No Magic for Me

Lisette Skeet

Strategic Book Publishing and Rights Co.

Strategic Book Publishing and Rights Co., LLC
USA | Singapore
www.sbpra.net

For information about special discounts for bulk purchases, please contact Strategic Book Publishing and Rights Co., LLC Special Sales, at bookorder@sbpra.net.

ISBN: 978-1-68235-609-8

For Your Courageous Self

DISCLAIMER

This book contains honest descriptions of a medically diagnosed illness from which I suffered. I describe its effects upon me and my recovery, which I achieved independently. In this, my second book about Myalgic Encephalomyelitis, I continue my account of the illness and the way it affected me for more than two and a half years until I found my way forward and was able to leave almost all the symptoms behind. It was arguably even more difficult to move on from the psychological damage caused to me by disbelievers.

My beliefs are informed by personal experience as well as research. The contents of this book, with my conclusions about the psychology that affects medical professionals and others, are the expression of my opinions with no assumption of medical training but my views are informed by personal experience, careful study and observation. I have undertaken a considerable amount of training in areas of counselling (especially psychodynamic theories) and psychology. Much was in an educational setting in college or university, where discussion and debate amongst tutors and learners was often invaluable.

The examination of aspects of psychology has led me to consider the mental processes that may affect the opinions of both the doctor and the layperson. My conclusions are drawn following careful consideration of unexpected and often quite extraordinary criticism, which occurred during the time I spent in a state of debilitation, and afterwards.

The implications and inferences that may be deduced from an examination of my method of achieving wellness may be open to question in the way of all scientific research. Any reader who determines to make every effort to bring themselves forward and away from chronic illness via the theories and ideas I've taken pains to describe, is free to consider the advisability of beginning their own research and seeking other opinions. This requires special note by anyone who has another, different disorder or disease accompanying their ME symptoms and which could bring its own effects, problems and needs.

PREFACE

A pony is a small horse, but a horse is not a pony!
Years ago, as a child who loved to read books about horses, I learned the above saying and I enjoyed pondering over it. Now, I believe the issue of myalgic encephalomyelitis (ME) compared with chronic fatigue syndrome (CFS) is similar. ME is a mighty challenge. CFS is comparable but it's likely to be a lesser evil.

This personal view of ME could be controversial; however, when I refer to the illness I had, I am definitely not talking about post viral fatigue. I believe that even chronic fatigue syndrome is significantly different from the condition which affected me, although a quick search online finds them linked (CFS/ME). In fact, my diagnosis was clear and as soon as it was delivered it seemed that everything (debilitating illness with repeated lapses and surrounding confusion) fell into place in many ways.

If a patient is as ill as I was, or as badly affected as another patient who has been diagnosed and lives with ME presently then, in my opinion, he or she has ME. If the illness presents minus many of the agonising symptoms (I list them below), then it is something different. That does not mean that a sufferer of chronic fatigue syndrome will not be interested in this history with my ideas, reflections and analysis, since it can be shown to be similar in some ways.

Therefore, my discussion of the condition known as Myalgic

Encephalomyelitis (ME) is specific. It isn't intended to define illnesses which are thought by some to be comparable *or* definitely similar. Nevertheless, ever since I recovered from ME there have been times in my life when a careful review of my diet has been beneficial, and my considered opinion is that the nutritional approach is a powerful starting point for many recovery programs, especially when it's addressed along with different aspects of personal care.

CONTENTS

Introduction

"A thousand knees, ten thousand years together
Naked Fasting upon a barren mountain
and still Winter, in storm perpetual
Could not move the gods to look that way thou wert"

W. Shakespeare

Poor me, poor you, poor us! Yes, of course. The mighty ME. What kind of description can ever come near the truth? For me, the inability to walk properly was one of the most frightening things that happened, and there were times when I could barely walk at all. I was in misery, even agony, and I was debilitated.

Some people will use similar adjectives or descriptions for an everyday headache. There's no reason why they may not and we all have our own frame of reference, but the difference in meaning is vast. The headache may have arisen after staring at a screen or driving home from work at the end of a long day. Not migraine, just a dull ache, it's uncomfortable and tiresome but the suffering is leagues away from being truly comparable with the many aspects of ME.

However, we must find courage. Crying is understandable but it doesn't help. The medical profession hasn't been able to step in and cure ME for over thirty years and even though I brought about a recovery for myself, I know the condition remains what it seems to be for so many: an impossible challenge. A neurological condition, some will say, but as long as I can manage it and feel well, I no longer concern myself with anyone else's absolute definition.

Writing about ME is hard. I know there are people who feel resentful, even angry when I address the issue of recovery via nutrition and self-help. This is saddening but I plough on because I want

1

to offer my ideas and some hope. I try to explain my recovery by that route. I'm not disingenuous. ME is awful, as we victims know and try to express. In reality, a change in your diet and complete overhaul of all you eat is not at all simplistic. It's very hard work indeed.

Following my effective return to good health, it seemed I would have to live without commenting about the fact that I once suffered from ME. Almost without exception, on the occasions when I made an effort to describe the experience I met with animosity from the listener. My survival and knowledge did not mean I would gain respect from others; the reverse, in fact, and I was essentially unable to help victims of the illness. Of course, I was not looking for glory but sometimes I would hear of a sad case history and torment myself over it.

When I learned that someone's friend had been diagnosed with ME, I felt a rising tide of fury when my informant came up with a surprised comment. "And *he* is a teacher!" (This comment does test my patience and resilience!)

For a long time, I never examined up-to-date theories about ME because I knew I would want to plunge into argument and, with justifiable expectations of being disbelieved it seemed impossible. Hearing of sufferers having a terrible time, I was distressed but felt powerless.

In an effort to protect myself, I consciously decided to be quiet and sadly it seemed essential, for there was a stigma attached to being identified as an ME victim. Far from being respected for my efforts, my recovery was supposed to have been spontaneous, my long months of debilitation a period of mental weakness.

Over years, I've had a multitude of experiences, some bad (including a foolish and damaging misdiagnosis of a different condition), some joyful (looking after my children) and of course many mundane. In the study of counselling theories and psychology I found myself on an interesting learning curve and began to reflect on my life.

When, at last, I consciously revisited memories of ME and paid attention to what the world is saying, I found that there is still terrific confusion and despair. Worst of all, is knowing that sufferers often reject a full-on nutritional approach for fear that it will add grist to the mill of suspicion. This makes no sense to me and I would like to explain why in this second book.

* * *

One day, half listening to a radio programme, I barely paid attention to it. I was getting on with some housework and the voices were a background noise. Topics changed from one to another and didn't hold my interest until the conversation focused on aspects of good health and the presenter talked about cigarette smoking and the harm caused by the habit. She raised the issue of finding ways to quit. Someone proposed a process without nicotine replacement aids of any kind, but their way was deemed too difficult. Many smokers would reject it. A psychologist explained that even if something is an estimable plan, it may be intolerable for another person.

When you have found a way forward, you will think your way is truly the right way!

He explained that, no matter how powerful one's ideas are, they should not be forced upon others because everyone has their own set of beliefs and habits.

I, too, reject the idea of force. It should be given no place in the treatment of illness and malaise. With regard to ME, most genuine sufferers know that being made to exercise will cause deeper exhaustion and lead to a prolonged set of symptoms which become increasingly hard to manage, with recovery looking less and less likely.

Studies of aspects of psychology led me to consider the possible mental processes that affect opinions about ME, whether they are held by medical professionals or other individuals including patients, their helpers, and the many who have no knowledge of the experience and therefore can only speculate. My conclusions are drawn following careful consideration of unexpected criticism, which occurred during and after the time I spent in a state of debilitation and was often extraordinarily hostile.

I offer my reflections respectfully, hoping they will strike a chord with readers. Inevitably, also, I still want to explain the discoveries I made and the ways in which I used them. My efforts to encourage others to try a similar path are genuine. And, as before, if you reject some of the things I say, you might still take an interest in a few and maybe there is value in the discussion.

Revisiting No Medals for ME

At around three o'clock in the morning on a Sunday in May 1987, just a few days ahead of the due date for my second baby, I woke with a start when I felt a sudden, single contraction. Mothers know that Braxton Hicks contractions can occur and be persistent near the end of pregnancy. They can seem quite strong but they are not painful, and once the process of giving birth begins then contractions are very obviously the real thing. I recognised the start of my labour, and for some hours I coped with regular pains at home, using breathing techniques. I felt excited and in control of the situation and yet, when I arrived at the hospital's maternity unit a little later, I was examined then turned away.

I was horrified! Couldn't I have a quiet room or a cubicle, where my labour could progress? No, the staff said. I should return home but, if I really didn't want to do that, I could go into the waiting room. I considered how it would feel to be forced to manage my pain amongst strangers without a nurse there to help me. I would feel embarrassed and overwhelmed. This meant I had to walk away from the hospital building, clamber into the passenger seat of the car, and tolerate (somehow) the drive along winding country roads back to our cottage.

"I won't put the car away!" My husband pulled into the side of the track at the front of our property.

"What happened?" A neighbour noticed my awkward struggle to climb out of the car. She followed us into the garden. "You look terribly worried!"

Midwives had decided I wasn't ready to be admitted to the maternity ward. I left the neighbour after explaining this. In the cottage, I made my way upstairs to lay on my bed, breathing carefully. Very scared, I was in a condition of shock but I was thankful that I could hear my mother-in-law chatting to my small son, telling him I was resting and he could carry on playing with his friends while she watched him.

I'm saddened by far more recent, similar experiences which have been related to me by mothers, since it seems the same thing happens nowadays. It's just a box ticking issue; the cervix has to be dilated a certain number of centimetres before the nursing team will identify active labour but it doesn't account for variations in different women, and it negates the purpose of a midwife, who should take on a nurturing, supportive role throughout the birth process.

In a way, I was lucky, because family doctors could be contacted on a Sunday in those days, and they would come when called. Before long, responding to an urgent call from my husband, our doctor came out to examine me. He then contacted the maternity unit, and I heard him engage in an angry conversation on the telephone, insisting upon my return to the hospital with as much haste as possible.

I was frightened when I entered the maternity ward this time, and shaking. It was a very different feeling from the confidence and courage I had possessed earlier in the day, and it was the result of the argument about my labour. Thankfully, I was not challenged again; instead, a young nurse made a comforting remark. "I think you're through the worst part!"

It was true. Contractions were almost over and, once I was established in the delivery room, the baby swiftly arrived.

When my baby boy was born, I was thrilled. A midwife remarked that I hadn't done things in the usual way. I noticed her comment and didn't much care, although I guessed she was covering her back, so to speak, or that of the team responsible for my distress earlier in the day. Now, all my attention was on my new baby and, once I was home again the following day, I settled into my new role as a mother of two little ones and assumed I could let the experience of giving birth slide away from my thoughts and be forgotten naturally.

* * *

At six years of age, Jonathan could do many things for himself. He liked to build models with Lego bricks which occupied him for long periods of time and, since it wasn't hard to care for my hungry new baby in all the ways I learned the first time around, my life seemed straightforward and I was happy. However, something seemed to be wrong with me and at first, it was hard to define exactly how I knew that. I kept breaking out in perspiration but it was early summer; the weather was fairly warm and I assumed my sudden sweats were due to being busy in some way. I thought it was odd that the episodes didn't seem to be triggered by any sense of pressure, nor was I aware of being especially overheated. I felt nauseous off and on, and sometimes I was dizzy.

By the time baby Andrew was about five months old I knew I was unwell but could only guess that a tendency to suffer from a viral sore throat seemed to be laying me low. The months passed with all the usual ups and downs of family life, and a thread of indefinable illness still bothered me. The Christmas period was difficult when I was often exhausted, and in the New Year I wondered how I could change this. I was very confused. I saw no good reason why I should feel ill, or give in to it! When I had some energy I used it, playing with my children or walking my dog. When I thought I was better, I went horse riding, but it was disastrous. I felt immensely breathless and stressed during the ride, and collapsed later that day into a state of utter debilitation.

At last, my local doctor listened to my fears. I had read of a weird condition called Yuppie Flu, I told him, and I had been trying to get strong and well for a long time, without success. Had I got Yuppie Flu? He was reluctant to comment but he agreed to refer me to a consultant.

Sure enough, I was declared a classic case. I had Myalgic Encephalomyelitis. What next? I wondered, sitting on a chair, marvelling along with the consultant over the complete absence of normal, healthy reflexes in my knees. I was advised that some people make a spontaneous recovery from ME. That was all. We left, myself and my husband, and went home, and except for that diagnosis nothing had changed.

I let my husband inform my wider family of my diagnosis. "They didn't say much about it," he told me after making a call to my parents. That evening, I received a call from one kind auntie, who listened to my description of the experience and asked if I felt better, in *any* way, for knowing I was really the victim of an identifiable illness. I wasn't sure. I think I felt stunned.

I have described the illness as it affected me, and in this second book I will list the symptoms again. Additional misery was caused by the attitudes of other people, and often they were unkind. I longed to recover and a sense of desperation began to grow, not least because I was frantic to continue to care for my children.

I joined the ME Association, and in those days my application began with a telephone call to a number my aunt found and gave me, and was followed up when I was sent an envelope full of leaflets and information. (My application wasn't online. I didn't even have a mobile phone in those days!) I seized upon the leaflets and accompanying letter, and read them carefully. At first, there seemed scant hope of recovery and yet one particular sentence played on my mind. It was a mixed message in a way, since it confirmed that the ME Association offered no route to a cure but recognised, nonetheless, that sufferers who make the most progress towards recovery have generally paid attention to their diet.

Then came a generous gift from Auntie Val. It was a parcel of books; some new, a couple well-thumbed, and they felt like a bundle of hope. I was struggling to read, but I went through them a few pages at a time and I began to develop some ideas and a plan. Drawing together the comment from the ME Association, and my aunt's kind gesture with her aim of offering help, I would try to make myself well.

I changed my diet and worked on getting better, and this is easy to write in a sentence and not at all easy to do. I began to make sure I ate breakfast every day, instead of skipping it or eating biscuits and drinking a cup of tea. A day or two of having porridge for breakfast began to show benefits, then I started to feel flat again and, when I delved into my books, I found it's best to avoid repetitive eating. So, I abandoned my porridge for a few days, and instead I would have a poached egg on toast, or a bowl of mixed fruits and a scone, or a cup of orange juice and some brown bread toasted and spread with honey. (To examine the reasons why it's best to avoid repetitive eating during illness, see the book I've referenced: Not All in the Mind by Dr Richard Mackarness.)

In my diary, I wrote the quote from Hippocrates.

Let food be thy medicine and medicine be thy food.

There was no doubt that my health and my ability to tolerate certain foods seemed to fluctuate for a time, and it was taxing to work out the way forward but I wouldn't give in. If I felt knocked back by a headache I really wasn't expecting, I checked my diaries, amended my diet and kept going.

I looked up the vitamins and minerals we need, learned what they can do for the human body, and became utterly convinced that it's essential to look at what happens in deficiency. In The Vitamins Explained Simply, there is an important sentence about being in need of more when an illness is present: ... *a sick person needs all the principal vitamins, but in daily dosages* larger than *a minimum maintenance dosage (page 124)*

It's clear from the same part of the text that when a vitamin deficiency has been ongoing, the corrective dose must be significantly larger compared with a maintenance dose.

There is a school of thought which insists that being inactive is partly the reason why ME victims lose their strength. In a well person, it's true that exercise in itself generates energy, but it's not the same for someone who is ill. The belief that so-called graded exercise will benefit ME sufferers is dangerous for them and yet it is proposed sometimes. However, to understand this, one either needs to be an ME sufferer who knows exactly how it feels to be pushed beyond the limitations of the illness, or someone who has deep compassion coupled with an intelligent awareness of the condition. When the symptoms are there, attempts to force an ME patient to be active creates awful weakness, can cause a dramatic relapse, and can only do harm. On a pathway to recovery, it's important to rest.

Having said that, with good nutrition bringing about a real change, it's useful to start to view the *possibility* of exercise with awareness of how it can benefit people and to begin to adopt a slightly different approach. Instead of setting oneself against exercise altogether, it's worth looking at ways to move forward. Certainly, in a condition of debilitation the requirement is rest and sleep, but one day, in a stronger condition that's genuine, exercise can be gentle and result in feeling better. I acknowledge that someone who has sat still or even been bedridden for a long time will have weak muscles, but once the nutritional cure is in place it should be reasonable to start gently moving about again.

I know there are ME sufferers who literally hide from sunshine because of weak eyesight, but the sun and fresh air are full of benefits. Even if the eyes are covered with dark glasses or a wrap, I'd urge anyone in this situation to raise their face to the sun sometimes. Staying indoors all the time is dreadful for mental health too.

Wrap up in scarves, have rugs over knees but do go outside. Too weak? Clasp a cup of hot soup and a wholemeal roll, and eat. Never, ever run on empty!

When I developed my theories about pulling all the strings, I was becoming sure of the importance of aiming for perfection in the care of oneself. I was determined to get well; I had to think laterally and my way isn't flippant.

I was successful, and after between two and three years of illness at last I regained my strength and shed all the pain and suffering. It was a strange experience! The world seemed different and my whole outlook altered because my mind felt fresher and my body felt as if it would work for me again. In a physical change that felt like a bonus, it was definitely a fact that my eyesight improved!

In No Medals for ME, I touched on how things were following my recovery, including what it felt like to stand amongst my wider family when they weren't interested in my health. There was significant mental and emotional harm, with attitudes still hurting and confusing me.

Years on, I realised that many effects of the harm never went away, not even with the publication of No Medals for ME in which I recounted my story, and recalled and considered much of what happened. An experience as a mature student in a university centre underlined the paucity of understanding of ME sufferers, and my extensive studies in psychology resulted in a multitude of thoughts and ideas.

THE GREAT STORM 1987

On a cold night in October 1987, I awoke because I could hear the sounds made by a terrific wind which was howling around the cottage. Baby Andrew was about five months old by that time. He was fidgeting in his cot near my bed and I lifted him out, to cuddle and breastfeed. I switched on a low lamp and sat on the side of the bed, taking care of the baby and listening to the noises made by the storm outside. Feeling unwell, I was still at the stage of thinking I had a prolonged virus of some kind. Often, I wasn't sure how I might explain my sense of malaise and only knew that I felt oddly weak.

Rain hammered against the bedroom windows. I remembered that the evening before, in a television weather forecast a presenter named Michael Fish suggested there would be no storm, saying "… a woman rang the BBC and said she heard there was a hurricane on the way!" To this, he added a remark no-one was ever going to let him forget. "Don't worry! There isn't!"

I had been awake for a few minutes when my husband stirred and then sat up with an exclamation. "Listen to that! It's like being in the middle of a tornado!"

The wind roared around the thatched roof of our cottage and I shuddered and drew my dressing gown around my shoulders with the baby tucked warmly inside. We were safe, we decided, in our recently renovated home but the lamplight suddenly went off.

When I peered through a window, there were no lights to be seen in houses around the village green.

The next morning, we still had no electricity supply and all our rooms were icy cold. The scene in that picturesque Suffolk village was different from the day before. From the front windows of our cottage, we could see the door of a telephone booth had been torn off and it lay on a grassy verge, and a nearby bungalow had a great hole in the roof where tiles were missing. Trees on the far side of the green had been flattened.

We lit a fire in the open hearth of the old cottage, and abandoned the normal routine of our weekdays. Six-year-old Jonathan was not sent to school. Instead, with his friends he was allowed to play outside, where the storm had passed and the children were excited by their changed landscape and unexpected freedom.

For me, the situation was grave as the day wore on, especially when darkness fell and I struggled to keep my children warm and also to care for myself with the various unpleasant ailments that had begun to plague me. I had not yet fully understood that I was being rejected for my physical weakness, and when I contacted my parents (who lived a few miles away and still had an electricity supply) to ask if we could go there, they said they were too busy to make arrangements for us all to visit them.

All over the country there was damage to property. Many trees had been blown down and some tragedies were reported. Around twenty people lost their lives. It was thought the disaster would have been greater if the storm had occurred during daylight hours.

It seemed the news team ended up with egg on their faces, especially as a later forecast had failed to offer a warning too. My understanding is that Mr Fish generally manfully insisted he told the truth as he knew it!

In those cold days my condition was developing and worsening, and it was inevitable that I felt extremely unwell. Compared to those who suffered consequences of the storm in more extreme ways, of course I was lucky.

Time passed. The power cuts lasted for several days but we coped, and my little boys were happy. I steadily became weaker and very confused by my persistent illness and unlooked-for restriction of my activities.

* * *

In that countrified place, young children gathered at a bus stop each weekday morning and waited with their parents there to watch them until the arrival of a minibus that would transport them to the local primary school about two miles away. I made my way painfully over the village green, walking with difficulty, as yet unaware that there would come a time when I could not cover the distance. The same little bus brought the children home at three o'clock each afternoon.

As we stood together, one mother told me people were gossiping, saying I had gained weight. Feeling the cold acutely, I had to layer my clothes and I certainly looked bulky. That spring, ten months after I gave birth to my second son and many weeks into being ill on a daily basis, I had at last begun to confront the fact that I was not recovering. I explained to my companion that I struggled to keep warm. I confided that I had read a news article, and was actually wondering if I had developed Yuppie Flu.

"Just because you read something" she retorted, "you don't need to think *you* have it!"

I was taken aback. Did she mean to speak in such a curt way? I wondered if she thought I was so silly, I chose to believe I was ill, grasping at a label without good reason. However, it was possible she intended to divert me from a potentially harmful train of thought. Maybe she simply had an unfortunate manner? I tried to ignore a sense of insult, hid my feelings and made no reply.

In fact, my fears couldn't be dismissed by this time and my analysis of my own situation was well under way. Where my symptoms clearly fell into line with a worrying possible prognosis it was impossible to pretend otherwise. With hindsight, it's easy to see that someone who chose to make me aware that I looked overweight, and argued against a growing concern which I'd confided, did *not* have kind intentions!

Let's Talk!

When I planned to write No Medals for ME, I saw a number of obstacles to the clear explanation of my situation and the points I wanted to make. I already knew that long descriptions of the ailments which can accompany the condition make listeners feel bored, lose interest and turn away. I could easily guess that my experience could be discarded, once read, since I'm not a doctor.

At last, I realised that I could certainly describe what happened to me. As long as I didn't affect more knowledge than I had, or become deliberately instructive instead of passing on my experiences and beliefs in a scrupulously honest way, I could hand on the anecdotes which are valuable to me and could be used to inspire another person with the very best of intentions. I now feel sure that the reader can choose how they see and respond to my messages, and there's always the option of sifting through the details and bringing thoughts into line with choices.

In my books, I offer the ideas and beliefs I found, used, and worked on. I can repeat assurances. For me, they were effective. Why not suspend disbelief, and ty them for yourself?

This is one imaginary conversation, but it involves some of the most typical questions that arise with relevance to my true history and my way of recovering from ME:

16

I really don't think a condition which has the potential to put me in a wheelchair, can be addressed by what I eat! What is all the research about, if that's the case?

I get it, absolutely. This is what I would answer:

I fail to understand why research into ME goes on and on when all the scientific knowledge is already there. Each vitamin deficiency results in an effect on the body (and the mind, too) and when someone is ill, they need more of those depleted vitamins. How is this being missed? It's extraordinary, and disastrous for so many people.

When I read detailed texts about the effect on the human body of a lapse in important vitamins, I started to spot similarities to some of my ME ailments. When I went on from there and examined the theory of masked food allergy, I saw more. I had nothing else to try, no medicine, no support and barely any sort of kindness coming my way. I felt like I was literally going to try to save my own life.

Even as I began to design the plan, I felt daunted. "Nothing will change or take away this monster!" My thoughts were against me, even as I tried to find a way forward. Yet, my way worked and I stopped thinking of the collection of ailments as one single foe, and saw them as signs that were directing me to look after myself.

So, I thought outside the box to the best of my ability. To review the above question, it's in two parts:

Can the condition be addressed by the nutritional approach?

Yes, I say.

Why all the research, then?

Why not simply let that be the case? Treat yourself as an individual. If others cannot help, you must do it!

If the nutritional recovery plan is complicated and clever, why wasn't No Medals more serious in its style?

In No Medals, I held at bay all the psychological analysis but I thought carefully. I was trying to reflect my experience in an honest way but there are important messages in the text. I described my approaches after I studied and the way my recovery unfolded, and I wanted to present my theories without over-complicating them.

I was truthful in describing my way forward, and as soon as any individual begins to examine the basics of good health, they will find there are dozens of related issues. Not only are vitamins and minerals important along with sunlight and fresh air, but all kinds of aspects which are relevant to the human system. With compassion for other victims, I wanted to offer something an ME patient could relate to, or partly, and I hoped I could bring ideas which others would like to try for themselves. I know, because I've been through the experience, that although exercise is generally important for everyone it simply must be treated with extreme caution for the ME sufferer. I looked to empathise with those in despair because they are mistrusted.

I added illustrations because I enjoyed creating them, and I was hoping to bring in highlights to some important points. A little dog? Her name was Sally. I longed to walk her again, and my longing was realised. A bowl of fruit? Eat healthily and well. A simple glass of water? Yes! Because keeping well hydrated really matters … and so on.

How did you get your shopping?

During the times when I was floored by ME, I depended upon my husband for collecting groceries. He did it, picking things up on his way home from work, getting the essentials. In the first months, I hardly cared what I ate, and concentrated on ensuring we were supplied with enough food for us all, including the things my children needed and enjoyed. Once I designed and developed my nutrition plan, my concern to get hold of foods which would provide my essential vitamins became far more acute.

Sometimes, it was painfully difficult. Once, my husband

instructed an employee to collect some items and my request for herbal tea was ignored or misunderstood, and caffeinated teabags were bought instead. Asking for a brown, seeded cottage loaf somehow got me a white, sliced one! I tried not to complain, and despite such muddles I gathered enough of the things I needed to start the recovery.

When I could walk with some strength again, keeping my balance at last, I could make my way across the grassy area in front of my cottage and take a short cut to the local shop. I could choose the things I particularly wanted to buy.

Unexpectedly, I found a friend in the shopkeeper who knew I had been unwell. She avoided commenting on the cause of my illness, but she was kind when she asked how I was feeling. I mentioned that I was beginning to be very careful about my food, and she shared her experience of migraine and said, often, the headaches she suffered could be traced back to a type of food. With a gesture and a rueful comment, she indicated a row of tinned soups.

"I can't have any of those!"

It was anecdotal but it was a truthful reflection of her experience, and it was in line with my discoveries about myself.

Seeing me outside the house, a new neighbour greeted me, introduced herself and began to be a helpful figure in my life. Rosemary was respectful and thoughtful, offered help with minding my lively two-year-old son, and told me I wasn't to worry about entertaining her. She would visit me sometimes, and help. The part she then played in my life was modest; she was a busy person with limited time to spare, and I had already suffered for many months. Nevertheless, her kindness was valuable.

Did you really have ME?

There is no question about it! I did. I developed ME in 1987 and suffered with the symptoms for many months. At first, like so many people, I couldn't identify any reason why I got so exhausted. I wasn't depressed or unhappy, loved caring for my children and pets, and lived in a lovely, countrified place. Repeated episodes of sore throat, feverishness, and bouts of cystitis were annoying, but I expected to recover and sometimes it seemed as if I was on my way to feeling better. I always believed I would progress, change and become well; then felt disappointed and unhappy when my physical condition deteriorated all over again. It took a long time to realise I was an ill person, and a great deal of reflection to mark that shocking birth experience as a possible fundamental trigger when I was reduced to utter exhaustion during painful stages of labour.

"I'm in my early thirties!" I was in despair. "Is this just the way I am, now?"

It seemed incredible that I was genuinely contemplating a life without the freedom to run around just as I always had before.

I tried to get on with normal activities and in the early months I didn't consider that I might need a specific diagnosis. Doctors dislike being faced with a patient who seems to have the flu' because it's a virus. It's unresponsive to antibiotics, and the usual advice to take painkillers and rest can be found without recourse to a surgery. Long before Covid-19 arrived as a serious threat in so many ways, every episode of cold or flu-like illness felt like a relatively minor nuisance which would surely pass, and yet episodes were so frequent.

There was no improvement and things got worse. Symptoms were nastier and I lost sleep at night, then suffered during the day. I shook sometimes, and walked awkwardly, even jerkily. In those days, it was common to read an article about ME and find the condition described as Yuppie Flu, a silly, derisive term which no-one wanted applied to them. However, the realisation that I must be suffering from that illness (no matter what one termed it) was gradually dawning on me.

Once I was diagnosed, there seemed little more to do for myself than sleep when I could and hope for a miracle, considering I was sent home with no medication of any kind. By the time my aunt sent books, and I tried to gather my resources with those snippets of information about creating a more likely scene for a recovery, my youngest son was two years old and I had been unwell for a long time.

Myalgic Encephalomyelitis: the real thing. How does one find the words to describe the awful ME? When someone else with an uncomfortable headache might describe it as terrible, but for the ME victim, the pain is off the scale? Sometimes, I could only drag myself from sofa to kitchen chair, and some experiences of being in that condition defy description. I felt cold and there was often confusion in my thoughts, or a dullness. Often, it seemed as if my once agile mind was blanketed in cottonwool.

Perhaps it's important to choose the words carefully. The English language is wonderful but people will say they feel awful, with a cold. So, how do you feel, with ME? Like hell? People say that with a sore throat or a hangover! It's tough because ME is worse than those things: far, far worse.

You were married. Why were you so lonely?
Why did my husband absent himself often, and seem to neglect me? I didn't want the obvious questions to stop me from writing the things that mattered. These stories are not about a marriage, as such. In truth, far more painful than loneliness was the cruelty I encountered. Spiteful comments aimed at someone who is already suffering aren't excusable and as a matter of fact, my husband didn't make them. However, I have a reflection that is relevant, and it's a small gesture in explanation.

My generation tended to try to stay in a marriage through difficult times. I thought one must maintain the family unit almost no matter what happened, and I had so much happiness in my family, finding contentment in being a mother. I was protected in many ways, since I wasn't forced to work outside the home. When I began a course of study in adult learning a few years ago (long after my husband left the family), I met a tutor in psychology, who surprised me when she announced to the class a personal belief which immediately struck me as questionable. She thought that women who stay in a problematic marriage and try to make it work, must be weak.

I must say, I was not the only older student who stared at her in astonishment. For a woman of my generation and upbringing, my choices were sensible. With the understanding I had of life, at the age of around thirty I was being brave. My brand of courage did keep me married then, and it also saw me through the times when I was bullied for my illness, by those who saw fit to do it. Somehow, I withstood their foolish hostility and insults, and if my self-belief wavered, it came back.

I don't care about food. It doesn't make any difference. As a matter of fact, I eat chocolate for breakfast, sometimes!
Comments such as this always make me feel sad. There is such potential for recovery via good nutrition and I hope you'll read the chapters I include in my books and consider a change of heart.

I'm not the only one who has suffered chronic symptoms and brought about a recovery, but some people will go part of the way towards accepting that a good diet might help, only to follow up with an argument, saying they already do the best they can. However, a normal diet for a well person isn't the same as the diet that's needed during times of illness. It's essential to look at what is important for each individual, and with ME there is a surge of need.

It's pointless to say, for example, *my partner eats the same diet as I do, and they are not ill.* This doesn't matter and it cannot negate the importance of the food eaten by you, the ME patient. Simply, another person's diet doesn't change your situation or needs. People differ.

What do you think ME actually is, then?

Following an initial illness and a period of time when the sufferer becomes physically (and sometimes emotionally) exhausted, there may be a depletion of essential vitamins. My understanding is that in times of physical and/or emotional stress, and during illness, a person needs more than the stated optimum amounts. There is an exception to be made where more can be harmful; this is true of some, and of course it's something to check by anyone who plans to increase their intake.

This genuinely scientific approach is absolutely blameless and does not remove the sufferer's right to be believed or treated fairly and well. Heart and diabetic patients (for instance) also do well to change their diet.

For reasons that are not understood (and I don't pretend to know them) the person who falls prey to ME might have a comparable life experience behind them to someone else, and that other person never becomes debilitated by it. In the quest for a recovery, I personally believe this conundrum shouldn't be allowed to make determination waver, nor put a block in anyone's way.

What if I try a nutritional plan and get really fed up with it?

Self-doubt creeps in, especially if a headache knocks you back and you can't account for it. We are susceptible to what we see others eating and enjoying, and to advertising, too. Sometimes, it will be natural to question the process, even feel annoyed about it.

Why am I doing this? I want to eat whatever I like!

In addition to the psychology surrounding food issues, there is a biological effect at play and in response to the sight of tempting food there are hormonal changes linking the brain and the gut, and resultant behaviour. There is plenty to research and study in this connection, and the brain is linked with behaviour and body weight.

Sometimes, once something is understood, one can restore faith and rescue the essential determination to see it through.

Some of these explanations are complicated! Have you any quick tips?

The bad news is, there is no quick fix. Having said that, the following notes may be very useful, especially if each and every recommendation is seen as part of the whole effort. In order to gain a better feeling overall, I'd suggest these ideas work best in conjunction with all the other nutritional and physical support structures which I describe in my Collapsed Puppet Theory. If you pull *all* the strings then each element of recovery, no matter how small and sensitive, works together with all the rest to support the whole plan.

Folic Acid I was sometimes confused by the way I kept on feeling like crying. I didn't want to cry! No-one knew I was doing it, and it only made me more unhappy. In my book about vitamins, I found a complicated but fascinating chapter on folic acid. I didn't try to diagnose myself with any particular anaemic condition but I considered there was sufficient information to direct me towards ensuring I had a better intake. I began to take a folic acid supplement as well as boosting my diet with fresh, deep green, leafy vegetables, and I found a definite beneficial effect.

Painkillers After I had worked through my understanding of how different foods affected me and made my diet as good as I could, I turned my attention to the fact that I was taking paracetamol regularly. I didn't take more than the permitted dosage but I began to consider that *every day* could be unwise. I gradually reduced the pills and then cut them out, and found that this created an improvement. Actually, it reduced the number of headaches I was getting. I know this can be seen as a debatable point, made all the more awkward when initially the body's response tends to be a headache! It's an unhappy, even confusing start, but if one allows the process another day or two, there can be a good result. For me, medication for pain relief was something I could phase out, and it helped.

I would note that I was once a personal assistant to a lady who was confined to a wheelchair, and she took liquid pain relief every day. For someone who has profoundly sensitive needs, of course, I would not recommend seeking the benefits of a change without a doctor's advice and support. A doctor who has the patient's best interests at heart could well be open to a discussion about this.

Sugars Sometimes, a snippet of information can be so valuable it should jump right up and be noticed. I hardly ever buy women's magazines these days but when I do, I often find that guidance about good food on health pages, is great! Over and over again, one finds advice is *not* to try to live off sugary foods and this is correct. It's because refined sugar can make you feel tired.

At a later date, a woman who was supposed to be supporting me was aware of my history of illness and recovery. She rejected the facts I described, and in sharp tones she declared a different belief. "If the body craves sugar, people should have sugar!"

Her freedom of choice didn't need to matter to me, although I noticed how harshly she spoke and I wondered why she seemed keen to contradict me, but I certainly didn't need to start questioning my method of recovery.

Craving sugar? When you are well, permit a little. When you are shaky with ME symptoms, and especially when they include that sense of needing to sleep deeply and helplessly all the time; truly, it's best avoided!

Fruit, vegetables, eggs (if you can eat them) Flood yourself with good things!

Take the ME sufferer who hasn't managed to achieve a real recovery. They find themselves in the confusing situation of feeling reasonable one day, and dreadful the next. They think they can use the energy that seems to be there, then they plunge back into illness and despair. Why do those highs and lows happen?

This is a typical experience of people who are developing the illness. Sadly, for some, they go on to be debilitated most of the time, although flu-like symptoms tend to disappear. I experienced this, especially after one memorable episode when I used my apparent energy to go horse riding. I really collapsed, that time. I went on to become increasingly debilitated, too. However, once I had established a better eating plan (by far), I was able to achieve a real recovery and my energy returned, was not illusory, and went on.

So, why do those highs and lows happen? The fact is, I don't know. I do know that it's possible to create a real difference which amounts to a recovery overall. I was determined to try a cure and I made myself as well as I could, and it was a more than satisfactory wellness.

Can you explain anything more about the Agony Aunt?

I protected the name of the lady who responded to my letter but perhaps it wasn't necessary. I have considered this carefully. Claire was fundamentally kind; of this, I'm sure. She was forthright and eloquent, and she was a well-respected person. She was perfectly certain of her point of view, and it's one that many people still consider to be valid but it's deeply upsetting for those who are ill with ME.

I wrote to ask for help and support. I wrote frankly, saying I was nearly mad with frustration at the loss of my freedom. I had often watched Claire on television and listened to her advice, and I felt she was someone I could trust. I certainly didn't intend anyone to think I had actually gone mad! Unfortunately, I had entered into a situation that could only add to my anguish.

She wrote back to me, and sending a handwritten letter was kindly meant but her words were harsh. Surely, she didn't realise how hurtful they were? She questioned my understanding of my situation. Had I thought *there may be a reason for the way I felt?* There was a world of meaning behind this question, and it wasn't in line with the truly physical nature of the condition. In fact, I answered that initial letter with a protest! I wrote to express my shock and underlined how active I normally was, when well. Her response came again, but only to say she believed she was right.

Even if you want to look at the helpful effects of a holistic approach, I am absolutely certain that no-one should tell an ill person they can actually recover from physical illness by altering their attitude! Fault, whether it's supposed to be the result of a poor attitude or foolish behaviour, shouldn't come into the picture and I maintain this even when disease results from actions. Undoubtedly, smoking cigarettes, drinking heavily or overeating will all cause harm to some people, but once someone has become ill there is no point in cruel remarks. Look at ways forward but don't *blame*.

I would think the responses I got from Claire reflected only a scant understanding of psychology. I don't think my case was considered carefully at all, especially as she unhesitatingly reflected a group perception which was typical at that time and has unfortunately persisted in many quarters. She stayed firmly within her own frame of reference and couldn't contemplate the possibility that I might be offering her a truthful report which could even have informed her usefully. Students of deeper aspects of psychology, especially those who study Freudian and related theories, would look to examine their own response very carefully, spot their lofty attitude and clarify their position both for themselves and the client.

Is it true that some people continue to question whether or not ME exists as a condition in its own right?

Yes, and it is part of the shock overall when victims begin to realise that they are ill *and* disbelieved. There are those, like Claire all that time ago, who insist on doubting there is even a condition which should be identified as ME.

In fact, there are various groups in terms of beliefs about ME.

It seems there are others who think the condition exists but cannot be treated?

The specialist who diagnosed my illness was in this group at the time. They are the medical professionals who understand and believe the condition deserves its label or designation, but tell patients they have absolutely nothing to suggest that's helpful. They may offer the slim hope that the illness will eventually resolve itself.

Isn't it true that some medical professionals do seem sure that research must go on, and that efforts to find more scientific reasons must be made?

There are medical professionals who are sure of this, and many sufferers too. They believe there can be no real chance of recovery from ME unless a medicine is developed. In this group, again there are those who acknowledge that some people simply recover spontaneously. However, they are looking for a medical cure and where they may be seen to differ from the above group, they believe the research needs to go on and is worthwhile.

Why would you think medical *professionals* are wrong?

I accept that the body of opinion which leads many sufferers and professionals to wait for a medical cure, is weighty and important. I know that research is extensive and genuine. For myself, however, I couldn't contemplate a future where I didn't take a hand in my aim to recover from ME.

I cannot explain the anomaly between the depth of scientific knowledge that exists in relation to human health and good nutrition, and the failure of the medical profession overall to use the information to its optimum effect. However, those who reject the recovery plan via nutrition may have a sense of protecting a set of long-held beliefs. Will they lose face if you begin to recover by yourself using nutrition and the support I described?

In that connection, will *you* think you lost face because you had something incurable and now you fixed it? Does that matter, if your energy returns and your skin glows and you can make life choices from now on? Does it matter what the world says, if you can walk? Do you care all that much what others think about ME, if you can make independent life choices from now on?

After being dismissed from the so-called specialist's surgery, I never returned to a general practitioner with a query about ME. As so many sufferers have found to their cost, one can meet with insulting treatment. The specialist had agreed that I must have ME, but, in itself, it was almost a useless outcome. I never pushed for a second consultation with him and I never gave doctors a chance to tell me that we all get tired, or I should try exercise to make me feel better, or pull my socks up and imagine a change of attitude would do the trick!

So, what more can you say?

After the publication of No Medals for ME I was asked questions. I reflected carefully and more memories were waiting to resurface. I realised, as they flooded in, that there had been far more unkindness demonstrated by others than I described; there were more symptoms than I retained in my conscious memory and in fact, since I studied counselling theories as well as aspects of psychology and methods of improving self-esteem, there was more to be said.

I remembered the full extent of the spite directed at me, and even episodes of real cruelty. Some memories had been deep within my unconscious mind, submerged, not hurting by being buried. They resurfaced and I visualised and heard, all over again, those people who turned against me with contempt, scorn, smug hilarity; certainty that such chronic illness couldn't happen to them. Hard words, mocking laughter and insults.

The sense of insult is dreadful. With dignity already threatened by the extent of the debilitation, the experience of feeling ill and also being criticised is unbearable. When I began to write this second book, I brainstormed at first and was affected by all the memories that had emerged after reviewing my own first effort. Many of them were still hard to bear, even after such a long time.

A Personal History

Childhood

One night in around 1968, my mother pounded up the stairs of our house in Essex, and rushed into the bedroom. My sister and I were asleep, but she shook us awake and made us sit up in the bed we shared because she wanted to see if we had head lice. She was in a terrible state of panic and her actions really gave me a fright. She didn't seem to understand that the infection was a common problem and blamed her friend whose daughter had probably picked up lice in school. The following day, inevitably, a special lotion was purchased and hastily applied to our hair. The treatment worked, but my mother's attitude and the whole episode made me feel very ashamed.

On that occasion, my sister shared my sudden rude awakening. As a general rule, it was I who was often made to feel awkward and somehow different. There was no outward reason for it and nothing in my childish behaviour to account for it. I was so very shy, I always tried to behave well so as not to attract a reprimand and yet, for reasons I cannot fathom, in a family where I had two sisters and a brother (none of whom produced the same response from our mother) I was sometimes made to feel unhappy. In some ways, I was even neglected.

What were the reasons for this? What makes a mother of three daughters treat one as the underdog? In times of illness, the additional suffering I endured as a result of a certain sense of being reproached along, often, with disinterest, was painful then and continues to seem odd, years on. Even after endless study of psychodynamic theories, it's unclear where the foundation lay in my family.

Chicken pox? As soon as I was no longer infectious, I had to return to school, and it was an all-girls grammar school where showers after games were taken in the nude and I was bullied for the livid spots all over my body.

Toothache? I was forced to visit a dentist who had no idea how to care for children and was irritable and rough, causing a phobia of dental surgeries which has lasted all my life. I was made to wear uncomfortable, ill-fitting caps on two front teeth for a time, which caused dreadful embarrassment especially as, again, I was sent to school.

Some of the traumatic times I suffered may be thought typical of a middle-class childhood in the sixties and early seventies, when parents were arguably less involved in their children's emotional responses to life events. Perhaps, in terms of the emotional side of the suffering, that's a valid point, and yet there was physical harm too. I was raised in a beautiful home surrounded by gardens, and there was every appearance of care and normality, but things were not always as they seemed to others. At the age of thirteen, a fall from a bicycle a resulted in a significant concussion but it wasn't identified until I had lain in my bed in a state of half-wakeful confusion, for a whole day.

So, the episodes went far in terms of feeling abusive. Now, in retrospect, they still look abusive, and there were times when I was treated in a way I'd never contemplate for my own daughter. Oddly, if I presented as debilitated, I always came in for ridicule and my mother tried to make it *not* the case if she could. So, I had to attend school as if I were not smothered in spots ... walk into a dental surgery trembling with fear ... wait it out, to see if my concussion was not affecting me after all.

I suffered a miscarriage at the age of twenty-nine. Barely nine weeks into my pregnancy, something went very wrong and I sadly lost that baby. I was shocked and grief stricken; it's a terrible time for a woman who is full of hopes and plans. Such things happen, and one must come to terms with them, although I think a mother never forgets that lost baby. Again, incredibly, I was treated as if I was odd. When my doctor sent me to the hospital, I called my mother (perhaps unwisely) but she wouldn't come to take care of my four-year-old son. He was sent to his other grandmother, where he was cherished and safe.

The next day, my husband collected me from the hospital and I returned home, relieved to be back with my little boy and my two amiable German Shepherd dogs.

In a brief call, my mother checked that I was at home. "It must be something to do with the other side!" she said. She meant, my husband's side of the family. "We don't have miscarriages."

Well, she hadn't had one. In fact, her sister, my aunt, knew the sorrow and shock of a miscarriage all too well.

All of this and more occurred within a framework of an apparently happy family, and my parents both adopted the same behaviour when I fell ill with ME. All over again, a sense of rejection during a time of vulnerability was an incredible thing to experience. The root cause of my treatment, of being thrust aside during a time of extreme need, was habitual and linked with that neglect when I was a child.

In fact, the steadfast kindness I continued to show my family was extraordinary and I still sometimes wonder if I ought to have separated myself completely!

I was thirty-one and my first child was five when we moved to a Suffolk village, where we lived in a picturesque thatched cottage for several years.

* * *

Adulthood

Soon after I gave birth to my second son in May 1987, I developed the nightmarish condition of Myalgic Encephalomyelitis. The reality began to hit me when I started to walk jerkily, and I couldn't raise my arms to a steering wheel, to drive my car.

"I can't go out and get my shopping!" I cried.

My mother's response was scathing. "If you stay like this, you can't do anything nice, either!"

It was an oddly detached observation; almost a warning, delivered just as if I had made a deliberate choice to remain unwell and debilitated. For what? Did she think I could get out of the situation easily? Her comment certainly wasn't anything to do with sympathy.

Unless one counts the fact that she was very beautiful, my mother had no reason to put on airs and imagine she was better than other people. We were not wealthy or titled. In childhood, my siblings and I were lucky to be generally healthy, and our home was a comfortable detached house set in lovely gardens, but our family was neither better than many others nor superior. However, my mother had a real problem with anything that affected me which she perceived as unusual or weak, and sometimes this was just silly, and sometimes it was downright dangerous.

It was a form of snobbery. *We don't get conditions that seem unusual ...*

It was saddening in those days, and of course such an attitude is out-of-line with modern attitudes (except, perhaps, in relation to ME). So, my history was of neglect and rejection when ill. I was seen as a nuisance when I was unwell or harmed, and I was not allowed to be a nuisance. Any suggestion that I might be needy resulted in challenge and often annoyance.

Because of a relative, the condition known as Multiple Sclerosis was always discussed with respect and automatic belief, but I never dared mention Myalgic Encephalomyelitis at the same time. My illness was ignored in order to make it possible for everyone else to live normally. It made me wonder: was I really an uncomfortable person to have around?

Slowly, ME began to be recognised as a condition by the rest of the world, and the rude phrase, Yuppie Flu, stopped being bandied about. Articles appeared in magazines, and my mother collected them. She then gave them to me, to read. I wondered what her point was! It was far too late to affect sympathy for my suffering, and providing poorly researched literature hardly helped, especially such a very long time after the worst was over.

If you see the family as something transient, where the parents let go as their adult children move on, perhaps you'll wonder why I labour these points. Some families split up once the children have become adults. People move away, decide to live abroad, or let irreconcilable differences lead to loss of contact. However, my mother did not let go and she very much wanted to be in touch with her grandchildren. I felt as if I was welcome in a way but only sometimes, and I remained more acceptable if I was not ill or sad. It was better if I concealed those things.

With the foundation of my life having been a tendency to make me feel different or in the wrong, it was no wonder I found myself at risk of going along with the idea that my illness was odd, when I developed ME.

THE SCIENTIFIC METHOD

At the age of eleven, in school I obediently followed my classmates into a classroom for our first science lesson. I had no idea what was ahead. We were confronted with long benches, high stools, Bunsen burners and a new teacher. There was a peculiar odour in the air. I wore the blue overall uncomfortably and, as it turned out, I truly hated the lesson. The teacher was certainly knowledgeable but he spoke English with a Polish accent I had never heard before and used words I struggled to understand, and I couldn't follow his instructions. To this day I am confounded by the high achievers in that class! Clever students, who somehow understood what to do, learned the subject and passed tests with high marks. We were pupils in an all-girls grammar school and expectations of our capabilities were very high.

I had been sent to the school because I passed the Eleven-Plus examination but the change from a tiny village primary to the much larger secondary school was utterly overwhelming. I hadn't the resources or the nerve to ask for the help I needed, and that was true in every lesson although where I felt happiest (English, French and Art) I muddled through more successfully. I was hopeless in Physics and Chemistry. I got the strings of my overall tied into a tight knot and always had to step into it instead of wrapping it around me. I burnt my hand and hid it, afraid to admit to the accident. I panicked often. Nothing indicated I would one day describe my mind as scientific, as I always failed any examination in this class! However, such things happen in school, especially to a shy child, and times change and bring different experiences and some revelations.

In No Medals for ME, I wrote that I have a scientific mind and in the informal sense it's true. My thinking is methodical and logical and I always strive for accuracy.

After a doctor who professed to be interested in ME gave me the most cursory of examinations, declared that I was a classic case and delivered himself of the casual comment that some people recover, I was left, high and dry, with nothing helpful from any doctor. I was disappointed and offended, especially as the consultant seemed to show a sense of excitement! (This was something to do with my case being typical in every way.) Afterwards, I never again consulted anyone in the medical profession about any of the symptoms.

I found my way forward after months of illness, and I was working from the evidence which pointed to the fact it is not a disease *process* as such. I learned about the vitamins and minerals in the human diet and what each one does for us, along with the importance of sunlight, and the awareness I gained by trial and error that helped me see, one cannot get rid of ME symptoms by fighting them. Exhaustion inevitably results.

I equipped myself to bring about a useful state of recovery and viable good health.

Crucially, I looked into what a deficiency of each vitamin can mean and found that some ME effects match those symptoms. Perhaps a blood test would not have shown up a deficiency? I don't know, because I kept away from the doctors who failed me. However, I have known other ME sufferers say they always test satisfactorily for indicators of health, and it's a fact which tends to make them believe there is little point in looking into a nutritional approach. Honestly, I think this is disastrous! Sending my intake up to maximum levels achieved a remarkable result overall and I remain convinced of the vital role the vitamins played in the process.

Years on from my recovery, I learned of the scientific diagram (this is readily found online). It can be applied to the method and the route I painfully developed for myself.

My Discoveries

Good nutrition is my main emphasis and I came to feel certain it is most important in making a recovery from ME. Add to the process every chance to rest, along with details like making the most of fresh air and sunshine, keeping well hydrated, and relaxing in bathwater at a comfortable temperature. Being so unwell and feeling anxious about what the future holds, does cause emotional vulnerability, so if there is any empathy to be found amongst family and friends then it can only do good to the sufferer.

I read the leaflets that were sent to me from the ME Association and this is the message I understood: there is no medical cure for the condition and some people remain ill for many years. However, *some people get well.*

How did they get well? I wondered, knowing for sure I wanted to be in that number. I learned that it was acknowledged the people who make a recovery are likely to be those who pay careful attention to their diet and lifestyle.

Scientific research into the value of vitamins and minerals has already been done. It doesn't lead to a single pill or a vaccination against ME but it does mean there is a mass of genuine knowledge to tap into.

Forgetfulness caused by poor liver function ...

Certainly, it's hard to let go of feeling the doctors owe you something but when it's possible to trace gems like this, surely, these are moments when the ME sufferer spots something important? Furthermore, it's a fact that this kind of detail sometimes turns up in the health and lifestyle section of any modern magazine.

Can I improve my liver function? How? This needs to be our next question, and so on.

People who are diagnosed, for example, with a fatty liver (which can be alcohol related, or it may not) often set to work to alter their diet, and the ME sufferer can do the same.

* * *

A Gentle Start

Perhaps it's sensible to begin making changes in a modest way, looking for simple ideas which will start to lay a foundation for a better picture overall. The lengths I went to may seem very challenging, especially while the effects of the illness are powerful.

How about drinking more water at first, and introducing two extra portions of fruit per day? To awaken your taste buds, make one of them something you may not have tried before: a mango perhaps, or a kiwi fruit, or a spoonful of prunes in apple juice. Try halving the amount of sugar you normally spoon into tea or over cereal; then think about changing your usual white bread to a wholemeal or seeded loaf, or go even more slowly and buy the kind of bread that's sold as half-and-half.

These things may be fractional changes at first, but as you interest yourself in your diet and its nutritional values you may feel small effects of such improvements and then, as strength returns, the effort becomes worthwhile and leads to interest in many more.

From these beginnings, perhaps you can build. Could you weaken your coffee and reduce the caffeine, or choose a decaffeinated option? Do you ever go hungry because nothing seems tasty? Whereas you may have been despondently not bothering to eat at lunchtime, how about warming a bowl of soup, adding a spoonful of grated cheese and eating a wholegrain roll along with it? Satisfying your appetite in a healthy way could give you a surprising boost.

Even a small upturn in your sense of wellbeing can encourage you to look for more ways to improve. Abandoning sugar-laden cakes could come next, and a piece of brown toast with honey might satisfy your sweet tooth in a healthier way. A glass of cloudy apple juice is one alternative to alcohol.

Before long, like me, you might consider aiming to get your diet as perfect as possible, making it so close to the ideal in your intake of vitamins and minerals, so free of damaging white sugar and even of caffeine, that you gain a real improvement in your energy and lose that ME pallor.

* * *

It does get harder ...

Making significant changes to one's diet can be traumatic. It is not an easy process and actually it requires courage. Venturing into the unknown as I carefully applied my research to myself, it was no wonder my heart quailed. I hoped for a good outcome and there was nothing else I could do to achieve one but I barely dared to think diet would tackle the monstrous suffering I was going through. However, I learned to abandon the sense that ME is a monster in itself. I came to understand that all the symptoms are a collective cry for help.

There were a multitude of difficulties when I began my route to wellness, and as I continued along the way. It's incredibly hard to let go of foods one perceives as comforting, and mine tended to be sweet things, perhaps partly because we ate home-made cakes and biscuits as children in my family. But sugars had to go, and although I missed eating chocolate, I was so sure I didn't want its ingredients (with sugar and caffeine) that I stuck to my diet.

Ever since those times, when I have a mild resurgence of familiar exhaustion the risk of slipping back into terrible illness is sufficiently frightening to make me redesign my nutritional approach and begin again.

VITAMINS

The Vitamins Explained Simply by Leonard Mervyn BSc PhD FRSC

This book was produced a long time ago but in its text each vitamin is described and the effects of deprivation detailed along with useful extra information and examples. It's no wonder I felt excited when I read it for the first time. I was hunting for answers, and there they were, leaping off the pages at me!

Those who are over-sensitive to light or glare, may be in need of Vitamin A (page 26)

Persons whose intake of thiamine is inadequate suffer from poor memory, lack of initiative, confused thinking and frequently from depression and fear (page 36)

A deficiency of folic acid can give rise to any of the following ailments: anaemia, diarrhoea, glossitis (inflammation of the tongue), gastro-intestinal disorders (more) (page 62)

A deficiency of biotin in man causes muscular pain, poor appetite, dry skin, a disturbed nervous system, lack of energy and sleeplessness (page 74)

One of the functions of Vitamin D is to release energy within the body (page 98)

I have taken these snippets of information at random from the book, and of course anyone who investigates its content (or a more

42

recent similar reference book, if preferred) may wish to withhold judgment until a consultation with a nutritionist can be had. I can only emphasise that it is full of useful notes along with detailed information to support them.

In Chapter 10 On Taking Vitamins, the author points out a quote from another source (Quigley) and writes: *Where a vitamin deficiency has existed over a long period of time, the dose that is given to correct the trouble must be several times larger than the maintenance dose (page 124)*

My story and beliefs are recounted on the basis that I am recalling and describing what I did, and explaining what I believe, and despite all the research I undertook I don't pretend to call myself a nutritionist as such. Nevertheless, I used intelligence, common sense and logic. If I am doubted, I don't mind about that, because my efforts got the results I wanted and made me well, although that's not to say I don't grieve for the lost opportunity of any ME victim who dismisses a nutritional cure out-of-hand.

I feel sure there will be ME sufferers who decide they'll seek the advice of a nutritionist before trying my way but I do suggest caution if you take your hopes to a person whom you trust because of their stated qualifications, only to find they try to sweep away all these theories without obviously giving them very careful consideration. Some people turn their face away from something important as a result of making assumptions. They may not be correct and you could be so discouraged that your *willing suspension of disbelief* disappears and your hopes get wrecked.

As I mentioned before, certainly it's important not to plunge into significant changes without medical advice if you have a specific condition alongside ME. For instance, asthma sufferers are sometimes affected in a specific way and undoubtedly need to look for extra advice and experienced guidance. This is also true, quite simply, if someone who contemplates making changes to their diet feels challenged and nervous. Nevertheless, I emphasise yet again that everyone has a right to question statements from medical or other trained practitioners where those statements could bring an untimely halt to brave and thoughtful efforts to recover from ME. If your care is a priority and your future good health is the aim, then any medical consultant or nutritionist should (at least) be open to a responsible examination of the vitamins route.

* * *

When I lived in Suffolk, I read an article in a local paper about another young woman who lived locally and like me, she had been diagnosed with ME. Needless to say, the condition was described as a mystery.

"She needs plenty of pills to help her get through each day," explained the writer of the article.

What kind of pills? I wondered. I took painkillers for the awful headaches, and the pains in the long muscles of my arms and legs. What else might the ME patient take? My thinking had begun to alter by the time I saw this article.

I began to realise that if addictive eating might be harmful, then so might painkillers, taken on a daily basis. I know this is a potentially contentious subject but, for me, this is what happened:

I took paracetamol. I wasn't exceeding the safe dose but, struggling with pain, I was taking the tablets most days. However, my careful approaches to good nutrition were getting me well, headaches were easing and, in a welcome change, they occurred less frequently. I wasn't slipping into the sort of acute pain in my head that had made me afraid. I wasn't hiding from bright sunlight, or unable to look at a television screen any more.

So, reducing the doses really slowly, I weaned myself off the paracetamol and yes, the headaches went away.

The Collapsed Puppet (Support)

During illness, my condition progressed beyond the apparent colds and infections until I lost most of my strength. Walking, I was jerky and slow. Trying to make a meal in my kitchen, I would drop items and fumble around. Once, I let a glass bottle fall from weak fingers and when it smashed, spilling milk, I wept because I hardly knew how to pick up the pieces and sort out the mess.

I had run out of resources. I felt weak and often shook. My thoughts were maddeningly foggy and pictures on a television screen, or words on a page, often just seemed to dance before my eyes. I began to think I resembled an abandoned puppet, with strings lying loosely around its collapsed figure. No-one was pulling me up and I had no chance (it seemed) of rescuing myself. However, I didn't want to give up. Slowly and painfully, I addressed the possibility of turning my situation around.

With the emergence of ideas and realisations as I read about vitamins and the effects of depletion, I began to consider that perhaps I did have resources. I made lists of the foods I thought might help my condition. I was hesitant, but I kept going. I added what I learned about poor hydration and planned to change my tendency to neglect ordinary water. Soon, I was considering how my days went, and I determined to alter the absolute status of victim. What else could I do for myself? Since I often lay on a sofa and simply shook, I started to attend to my personal comfort.

Cold? I dragged myself up to get an extra jumper.

Overheated? Lying in a bath full of water at a moderate temperature was helpful.

Miserable inside the house? I didn't force myself outside on a cold day, except when I couldn't avoid it. Sunshine provides both comfort and warmth, so when the weather was fine, I managed to step outside and sat on a chair with my face lifted to the sunshine.

So, this is about gathering together everything you can think of, everything that might be beneficial. Don't ignore small hopes, add them to your efforts, bring things together in the process and make it work.

While you are very ill with ME symptoms, it seems unlikely that a feeling of wellbeing will ever return. You long for good health to be restored, with that debilitation in mind and body gone, and your distress and pain banished.

Physically, in terms of activity, I'd say, don't ever drive yourself on. No-one must try to tell you this is a good idea because, the fact is, if it's ME that afflicts you, you will get worse. The symptoms will crowd in and multiply. The very best way forward is to provide yourself with optimum nutrition.

I changed my thinking and instead of envisaging an invisible foe called ME I saw this differently and understood that the groups of symptoms are produced by the body and system in a cry for help. Since this offers a powerful alert to a fundamental problem, it's logical to believe therefore, the body is truly working to save and protect the sufferer.

So, I think it's important not to imagine there's a fight against *yourself*. Try not to see the body as an enemy! Instead, look for comfort, and do it the right way.

This plan is about pulling all the strings, thinking of everything and leaving nothing aside if it could possibly bring some benefit. Think of the strongest, most important string being connected to good nutrition, then imagine you are pulling some more delicate strands. Comfort, as described. Personal care, so your face feels fresh and your teeth are clean, and your hair is brushed and tidy. To achieve good hydration, you can make water more interesting with fruit juice or herbal tea.

It's vital to seek the best level of peace of mind you can, so leave aside watching stressful television programs or taking on board someone else's difficulties. Perhaps you see yourself as a compassionate person, but you need to nurture yourself when you are debilitated.

Have the sleep you need, but if you cannot sleep at night, know that resting in bed, relaxing and breathing quietly, will help you to a great extent. Breathing techniques can be really useful to achieve such relaxation. I like to close my eyes, imagine each part of myself starting at the top of my head, and believe I am completely relaxing. Just imagine … one thing at a time … and slip into a peaceful state. So, one of the strings being pulled to hoist you up, is a sense that you are peaceful and that peace brings some comfort, and that comfort brings a little more strength.

The Beautiful Racehorse
(Appropriate Care)

It's stating the obvious, but humans are made of flesh and blood and it can be astonishing how they forget that important fact! Whether someone smokes cigarettes, drinks an excess of alcohol or take drugs, so often they harm themselves. Perhaps an ME sufferer does none of those things and really feels like protesting, saying they are doing their best. But now, the aim is absolutely optimum self-care and it could be time to question old habits.

Because of that *taking care of flesh and blood* analogy, consider how you might start to care for a lovely animal, which has been placed into your care. It is valuable and needs to be kept in optimum condition. You wouldn't neglect it. You wouldn't feed it on inappropriate foods, or leave it to become thirsty. Then imagine you are comparable to a racehorse! Take care of yourself with great food, plenty of clean water, and the surroundings and comfort you need. Give yourself the same kind of respect which you might have for a creature which depends on you for all its needs.

Learn to value and respect yourself. Being ill isn't your fault. You matter, and you deserve the very best care, even if you have to provide it for yourself! If you are unlucky, as I was, and the feeling that you are beaten down emotionally is hurting you, gather strength from personal self-belief. If you have kind people around you, then value them too, because they will help you to feel brave.

Discouraged

During the period of recovery, there may come a setback. A nasty headache seems to hit you from nowhere, or maybe there's a shocking return of some of the symptoms. At such times, life looks bleak, the temptation to question the process of self-healing is huge, and simply hiding and falling asleep feels more tempting than staying on the pathway via nutrition.

Do rest, of course. Then, gather your courage. When you are able to pick up a pen (or open a document on a computer) write out your diet diary and reflections. Once the mists have cleared a little, you might be able to trace some kind of pattern to the relapses. Did you get too confident, and overdo the physical activity on those days? Did a headache develop after eating a particular food, and has it happened in just the same way before (since you began to work on the diet)?

Be kind to yourself. Rest, doze and drift, keep warm (or cool, depending on the vagaries of the condition). Never, ever let someone tell you that you must get moving. Hang on to hope and keep trying.

* * *

It's clear by now, that I don't want to call the recovery plan a fight. The important thing to recognise, is that ME symptoms are alerting the sufferer to aspects of the condition. They are indicators. It's possible to work to correct one's state of health and bring it back to a bearable, even a happy state. So, there's no battle; instead, the recovery is about working hard to help and support oneself.

When you take a hand in your own care, honesty is vital. Perhaps the vitamins issue seems tiresome? It's tempting to reject the whole idea and you firmly believe you have enough of all groups of foods. Perhaps a nutritionist has even said so. I'm not trying to put any qualified professional down but the fact is, there is more to it when you have ME. There's more than just following recommended guidelines, and actual learned experience is valuable and real. A simple example might be as follows.

Consume more Vitamin C, you tell me? Well, I ate a tomato, today!

Did you, for sure? Or did you just have a couple of slices of tomato on the side of a plate of food which, as a matter of fact, you then pushed away, half eaten?

How about trying this for your lunch? Two whole tomatoes, sliced, grilled or lightly fried in a little olive oil, and placed on top of a couple of slices of wholegrain toast. Adding a grilled or fried sardine will make the meal tasty, and give you protein. Drink the juice of a freshly squeezed orange alongside this small meal and you will really boost the intake of Vitamin C.

We can fool ourselves in some significant ways, especially where a behaviour is cherished and fondly thought to be helpful. Regularly drinking more than the recommended daily amount of wine or other alcohol in order to relax is a typical example of behaviour which is born of seeking comfort but actually does harm.

Take the heavy drinker who suffers frequent migraine headaches and insists they are due to stress. The consumption of a whole bottle of wine most nights cannot be dismissed as a factor in the headaches. The drinker is battling against the body's needs, not supporting them.

Argument for
Argument's Sake

Everyone has a right to their own point of view, and also the right to express their thoughts. However, they may be relatively uninformed and this can be true even when they feel sure of their ground. Perhaps their life experiences have never shown them the things you know, or maybe their education (at any level) didn't cover the issues in question. In intelligent discussion, where participants are willing to listen with open minds and share their thoughts and ideas, everyone can benefit and no-one needs to become defensive, upset or angry and no-one should feel belittled.

Sometimes, an individual's argument is nothing but deliberately awkward and the only sensible thing to do is ignore it. Argument with no foundation or point needn't be offensive in reality, since it's probably harmless and in that case, it doesn't matter and you can rise above it. Nevertheless, if you are really struggling with the comments made by another person it may be helpful to reflect on how this happens.

In a gathering with a group of women, I had a growing awareness that they were being lofty. It began when we talked about holidays.

Why was I so suntanned? I was asked by one, who hadn't seen me for a long time. Had I been abroad?

I knew my face was brown and freckled. I explained that I had been exercising a collection of dogs, including a couple of spaniels belonging to a friend and my own terrier. We went out almost every day, I said, going on to add that summer time in Essex that year had been lovely. I liked to head for a recreation ground where the dogs raced one another while I walked around its perimeter. Sometimes, I took a picnic and made myself comfortable on a rug spread over a grassy mound. The dogs made their excursions away from me, then rushed back to share my sandwich crusts, and I watched them and enjoyed the sun and air. Those were happy times!

My companions commenced a strangely pointless argument.

"We *haven't* had a nice summer!" said one.

Another agreed. "No, the weather's been awful in this country! I went to Spain ..."

So, what happened? I was telling the absolute truth and yet I was supposed to be wrong! I was shamelessly contradicted. This has its foundation in habit, and I was with people who rather liked to affect superiority (although this was only their perception). On that occasion, it might have had something to do with envy. Simply by wandering around the Essex countryside, spending nothing on foreign travel, I ended up looking relaxed and well! The suntan in itself bore out my side of the argument, had I chosen to keep it going, but there was no need for me to perpetuate it.

Unkind people can't generally spoil happy memories, and I cherished my thoughts of those peaceful hours, when I sat on the grass with my face warmed by sunshine and animal companions around me.

* * *

Wonderful though the English language is, there are limitations in describing ME. This is because we use the same collection of emphatic terms for different ailments. Certainly, a headache can be very painful; a bout of sickness makes the victim miserable; a sprained muscle is sore. Since such things are often described, variously, as (for instance) *torture* or *ghastly* or *agony,* this diminishes our ability to fully explain our illness. Furthermore, as a migraine sufferer myself, I would even go along with identifying it as something like torture! Yet, in a bout of ME sometimes I would get a migraine *and* a number of other symptoms all at once.

So, what can one do to create accurate descriptions? Always assuming someone is prepared to listen, since the most elaborate words available may not hold the attention of others!

I remember, if someone actually asked about my health, I felt real longing to detail exactly what was happening to me! I wanted to explain the many symptoms and how it felt to be so debilitated. There were times when I could barely speak, but on the occasions when strength was fractionally better, I might attempt my description. I think I always hoped for a listener, but no matter how kind the initial question seemed, in moments, I saw them lose interest, avoid making eye contact, turn away and yes, in the most unhappy of such situations, they looked doubtful. The list was just too long.

* * *

Debilitating, pride wrecking, life-changing ailments.

"Starting from the top ..." I used to think, "the suffering goes right through me. My head aches, my mind feels fuzzy, my eyes are sore ... There is something wrong with every bit of me, all the way down to my feet, which seem to have gone limp!"

Headache. Sore eyes and poor eyesight. Nasal congestion. Sore throat. Stiff neck. Shortness of breath. Aching joints. Racing heart. Upset stomach. Cystitis. Weak muscles. Awkwardness and difficulty in moving, even jerkiness. Flushing skin alternating with cold skin. Fatigue. Confusion. Memory loss. Poor concentration.

Often, I was literally crawling instead of getting up and walking properly. I was flooded with oddly cold sensations but, sometimes, I was strangely overheated. I couldn't clear my fogged thoughts. It was impossible to exercise without feeling much worse and very weak, and I realised that forcing myself forward was a disastrous idea.

I'm deeply compassionate towards anyone who has ME and has been asked to try to tackle graded exercise. As for being asked to show someone you can run (it does happen), just say *no!*

* * *

Some people are not simply being thoughtless when they argue against another's experiences. Sadly, they intend to be unkind.

From May 1987, I struggled with bouts of illness for many months and they seemed to be viral. I often had a sore throat, and suffered from fevers, episodes of cystitis, headaches and tiredness. I felt more and more worried as time went on and I couldn't leave those persistent symptoms behind. I probably made light of it in general, and as a rule I was an independent person who wouldn't have expected others to interest themselves in my health. However, once the condition had really floored me, I was very ill indeed and there was no possibility of affecting normal strength. Weakness and debilitation affected me, and I was vulnerable.

Even following a consultation and medical diagnosis, my condition seemed to dent the consciousness of very few people, and only one relative called to offer her kind interest and support. Some of the people who had mattered most in my life up until that time, stayed away as much as they could.

Most people will naturally look for some sort of explanation for rebuffs. With ME, victims feel emotionally sensitive, as if many layers of protection have been peeled off and it's exceptionally cruel to be forced to justify perceived weakness. Someone who is ill long-term can lose masses of self-confidence and that's inevitable, especially when the condition isn't understood. He or she really is going to wonder what they did to deserve unkind remarks. It's often apparent that one has attracted unwelcome distrust, and the impact on a person who is already miserable and confused simply cannot be fully described. Who is entitled to sigh and shrug about someone who is ill, or even mock them?

In order to make a point about how odd they think ME is, disbelievers commonly try to suggest it is unlikely to affect *erudite* people! This is an unacceptable train of thought! Does the multiple sclerosis patient fit a certain intellectual category? Of course not. So, why would anyone adopt a scornful attitude towards the ME patient?

Looking back, it becomes clear that hurtful words were something that did the most damage to my peace of mind, and my natural resilience was diminished. I had every wish to return to the outdoor activities I loved as well as enjoying every aspect of being a mother, and I simply couldn't bear to hear anyone suggest I chose to be ill. I began to wonder why anyone would kick someone who is already down? It seemed baffling and yet, in a set of memories, I realised that cruelty and bullying were consistent with aspects of my childhood.

Was it wrong to want some help? Who refuses to support a family member? Following my recovery, I made up my mind not to ask anyone for anything, ever! I had learned a hurtful lesson. But cruel comments felt worse than inaction and the old adage of saying nothing if you have nothing kind to say, really does apply to treatment of an ME victim.

I've been asked why I don't reflect bitterly on my ex-husband. Certainly, he had no idea what to do, and chose to try to carry on almost as if he lived alone (incredible, when you consider there were children there!). In fact, he did nothing that was actually damaging. I can't remember any unkind words. He went to work every day, collected shopping (with a fine disregard for the specific things I requested, generally!) and simply reflected an absolute inability to see anything more than the diagnosis and that chilling fact that there isn't a medical cure. And after all, he wasn't the only person to react in that way.

When I got well, I overheard him in a telephone conversation and he was telling a work colleague that the worst seemed to be over.

"She's better!" He assumed a long-suffering air which could have been maddening, but I knew he was trying to bring things back into his frame of reference, and his more typical humorous and kindly ways. "She wants to get going," he went on, and it was true. I did!

Perhaps we should get really tough and say, think about any ailment that is terrible, and you know it is and you fear it. Would you try to demean or diminish the potential for misery in someone who contracted it? No? Why is the ME sufferer different? Why isn't she entitled to the same respect? Many people rejected me, criticising me when I was down, even though I had never been dully depressed or without courage before.

Disbelief often stems from fear and in fact, they were the ones who lacked courage. What is the root cause of their fear? It's a feeling of weakness, they aren't able to address your problems so they project that characteristic onto you. In fact, I was very strong.

There should never be a fight to be believed. Nor should there be any question about being valued when you are ill, regardless of its cause. No one would suggest you were being ineffectual if you broke your leg and rested up. *You broke your leg? Of course, you have to take care! Of course, you were not to blame.*

Sometimes a casual remark is obviously foolish and yet it absolutely cuts to the quick and only another ME victim could understand the reason why. It seems incredible when some people remain determined to reject the difference between ME and ailments which are certainly unpleasant but come nowhere near it in terms of misery. Migraine is one example. A dreadfully painful condition, it often brings sickness, sleepiness and debilitation too. Yet it can form just a part of the overall picture for the ME sufferer. In a deliberate rebuttal of my attempts to describe my suffering, one person highlighted their perception of another's chest infection and pointed out, they were brave (with obvious implication that I was not.) I'm sure they were brave. I'm sure it was not nice, and I wouldn't be kind if I belittled it. In an older or weakened person, a chest infection is quite dangerous, but … how long did it last? Not years!

However, this type of argument is designed to make it easier for a listener to brush off the enormity of the ME experience, finding excuses for past dismissive behaviour and reasons for its perpetuation.

* * *

As an aside, there is a condition known as tinnitus which is characterized by persistent ringing sounds in the ears. Anyone who has suffered from this problem knows it's all too real. It might simply be annoying for some, but it drives others to despair.

Commonly, people who do not suffer from this condition will propose that it's just the perception of the sufferer and they aren't really hearing actual sounds; even mooting the possibility that they are mentally unwell. It's an offensive suggestion.

People who become ill have a right to be respected and cared for, no matter how their illness came about.

When a dear relative passed away, there was censure because he was an alcoholic and I was shocked to hear the presiding vicar make reference to his addiction during her eulogy. Many of the faces that turned to one another in sanctimonious agreement were those of the kind of middle-class drinkers who could be very challenged themselves, to give it up.

* * *

Here's a remembered conversation which many sufferers will recognise. When the telephone rang, the call was welcome. I was very lonely and it would have cheered me to listen to my mother chat, telling me her news, bringing a little normality into my day. Instead, beginning with a reasonable question, the conversation was very short and almost instantly I understood that the question was a challenge.

"How are you, now?"

Could I offer something of my anguish? I had no strength for proper sentences but I managed a few words. "Not better … struggling."

"Oh, for heavens' sake!" The retort came fast. (Why did I even hope for something kinder?) "Can't the doctor give you something? Some sort of tonic?"

Impatient, disbelieving and unkind, she didn't care what that "something" might be. Anything to stop me complaining that I was ill. I, too, would have clutched at the offer of medication (had that ever been forthcoming) but my reason was my vulnerability and need. Her reason was certainly to make me less needy but her implication was that I was malingering.

"No," I had to say. "There's nothing." Weakly, I replaced the receiver. There were tears that time, and I felt very afraid for myself and my future.

On a different occasion, still only in a telephone call since I was generally kept at arm's length so to speak, she seemed to throw me an unexpected lifeline. "I have thought of you coming to live here …"

I would have set aside all my hurt feelings for the sake of my little boys, knowing they would have good meals and a home which had many bedrooms and a huge garden. A cleaner came weekly to ensure the house was cared for, and I would have been conscientious about my behaviour as a guest, and that of my children.

My heart rose. "Oh! That would be …"

She interrupted me swiftly, following her train of thought and bringing it to an end. "It probably wouldn't work though." There was a pause, then my hopes were dashed. "No, I don't think it would be a good idea!"

It was a cruel thing to do, teasing my mind with a possibility of some relief, then rejecting any chance at all of my acceptance. I don't know why anyone would think aloud about something which clearly wasn't really an offer of help, when the desperation of a daughter was so great.

Nowadays, people talk about clinical depression with respect, even a sort of reverence in a swing from old attitudes. It's the right thing to do, when the misery of depression can lead to the worst of outcomes for someone who finds no joy in life and really needs all the support they can get. Why not respect the ME victim, who cannot help but feel miserable about their limited life? There's a strong contrast between the comments people make about depression compared with the things they say about ME.

I know someone who is very depressed … it has been a struggle … he can be proud!

I know someone who has ME … it's a mystery condition, and a lot of people say it's all in the mind …

On a very simple, surface level, perhaps the consideration that most people simply don't understand how it feels to be afflicted with ME could help in coping with their rudeness. However, the unhappiness which some sufferers have expressed to me at times does seem to underline the fact that this is not enough. Even if that person who confronts them is baffled, with no idea what to say or what can be done to help, why not be kind?

As that ill person, once you realise you are suspected of malingering you have an almost impossible task. It is better not to show your anger, your sense of upset, indignation or fear because you will be labelled a misery. How hard it is! You have to be doubly strong. Stick to the truth (why shouldn't you?) but unless you are very lucky with helpers, you will probably feel you almost can't show the pain.

Some people withdraw, or they may even try to be hurtful to make you feel less of a bother. They are challenged; they don't want to feel forced to wonder what you have or how they might play a part to help with management and recovery.

A PSYCHODYNAMIC PERSPECTIVE

Many thoughts arose from writing No Medals for ME and they were painful, subjective thoughts. They belong to me, as personal reflections which it would be impossible to convey in full, especially to those who knew me and thought things were otherwise. My experiences, and my interpretation of them, don't negate the experiences or memories of those who knew me, although differences of opinion in recollection always have potential to be contentious and that's the way of families. I had to reassess my life and in doing so I recalled and reviewed a somewhat odd childhood.

I set aside analysis when I wrote No Medals, looking at the suffering I went through and the means of my recovery. I wrote about being disbelieved in a factual way, noting that it caused confusion, but emotions like disappointment and incredulity, even anger, affected me as a result of the perceptions and behaviour of others.

In a serious analysis and deeper reflection, plundering the memory to examine old hurts is painful all over again. If something was dreadful years ago, it gets no more bearable after time has passed by and often stays dreadful despite a better understanding of how it came about. When ME developed and affected me, and especially during the many months when I was confused as a result, a certain spitefulness from some of the people around me was renewed. It had been there before but it was shocking to realise and remember that it had always happened.

Again, thinking about those comments, many of which were knowingly unkind, I go through a process: the sense of shock along with incredulity, swiftly followed by hurt and even, for goodness' sake, self-blame. Why do I deserve all this? I wondered, and I felt fearful of the future. I was only human! During my review, I even found myself pondering over the possibility that I actually scared potential helpers away!

Since then, I have studied many aspects of psychology and I know now that some theories can be applied to create and broaden an understanding of what was happening. If that understanding doesn't help with the painful thoughts and responses to others who aren't kind, nevertheless it provides some kind of support. I think one develops a set of cushioning reflections based on that better understanding as they help with developing self-esteem. Eventually, an acutely sensitive, hurt reaction disappears.

Pack Mentality

In relation to ME there are some tired old phrases around. I detest them all.

A little-known condition ...

A mystery illness ...

It's easier to copy and use these phrases for anyone (be they a medical professional or a layperson) as opposed to making huge efforts to work out what might be happening to an ME patient. The words have been quoted too many times and the ideas are brought forth and transferred again, to the next victim. Those who pick up and run with the old nonsense create a block to the obvious fact that human beings are made of flesh and blood. We need to look after ourselves, sometimes far more intensively than we realise.

A pack can be just two people but it can also consist of many more. A group can be whipped up into a mindset of unbearable cruelty at its worst, often resulting in thoughts or actions which each individual might not demonstrate on their own. Behind that individual who confounds you by frowning and being suspicious are all the invisible influences. Quite literally, they are copying each other. Perhaps they will even say something like *I heard that it's all in the mind, and gets worse when people keep worrying about it instead of getting out and about!*

They aren't discerning, thinking themselves clever when they buy into the myths but in fact they are not clever enough to spot their own weak behaviour which is a block to an independent view. I have quoted a long-ago agony aunt, who simply repeated a few silly things she had read. She brushed me off, wrote that I should look for a reason for the way I felt, considered I was depressed even though I had a consultant's diagnosis of ME and was well able to clarify my feelings. I wasn't depressed and in that, I was lucky. Neither clinical or post-natal depression, nor even a simpler sense of feeling tired of the way things are, were ever my problem. I longed to be active and free from pain. Lofty treatment has nasty effects, and it's also disgraceful.

Some attitudes are imponderable, regardless of theories! Why don't people view multiple sclerosis with animosity and disbelief? Why don't they disrespect motor neurone disease? Those conditions seem more real? How real is ME, when someone is unable to walk or talk?

It's sometimes stated that some sufferers look well, but I have never seen a victim of the real thing (ME as opposed to post viral fatigue or even chronic fatigue syndrome) who hadn't the typical white face, often referred to as *pallor*.

Transference and Counter Transference

It seems modern doctors will generally acknowledge the existence of ME and its associated health issues. Outright disbelief in the problems the patient reports may be far less common than it was thirty years ago. However, they still tend to say there isn't anything to be done to achieve a cure. These remarks are connected with transference, bringing commonly held beliefs and comments into the picture whereas in fact the nutritional route is likely to create a wonderful outcome.

I couldn't treat the last ME patient and I can't help you! This could be the basis of their response, no matter what you have researched for yourself and would like to try. Doctors are rejecting something they haven't been trained to deal with, and they aren't willing to equip themselves with extra knowledge, even though detailed information about vitamins and the effects of depletion is readily available.

General practitioners appear to confuse ME with chronic fatigue syndrome, but the symptoms of ME (the real thing) are far more varied and far worse than exhaustion alone, unpleasant though it is.

Why is it that some people are so against your brave determination to get well? We know most doctors do their best for us but what makes them (or anyone else) want to purse their lips and shake their heads, wrecking your resolve and seeming to put you down? It's useful to see their resistance as their own problem since there may be a form of self-interest at play.

People who reject the proposal that recovery can be achieved via nutrition are looking to protect something (or unconsciously protecting something), and the root cause of this attitude is worth questioning. What are their interests? Are they afraid or perhaps too lofty to be drawn into a situation which might rock the foundations of their beliefs, and even teach them something? It could be that it feels much easier to follow the course one always took and fail to question it and this is especially true of medical people who have trained extensively, although they have every duty to listen to new ideas too.

Transference

Theory In all our life experiences, there are lessons to be learned and some of them we identify, and talk about and consciously remember. Some, we pick up on an unconscious level and when this happens, they can be buried deep beneath our surface thoughts. However, they do affect our thoughts and behaviour. In a psychological process called Transference, the responses and resultant actions which we have already adopted can resurface and make our behaviour the same, all over again.

People in general People who have dominant and manipulative tendencies could learn an early lesson, which is that they can force others to do their bidding if they use certain tactics such as charm, threat or another approach. Those with submissive tendencies will learn that they feel safest if they go along with the bidding of others, even when the situation feels unfair. People fall into patterns of behaviour which, without psychodynamic counselling which helps them to identify those patterns they become regular and habitual and unchanging. These patterns are particularly harmful in a relationship where there is an unequal balance of power, even abusive, but they can also be found occurring between two people who are essentially unknown to one another

Theoretical example (doctor and patient or tutor and student) The professional person is so used to being believed and obeyed, they forget they could be challenged and doubt they could be wrong. In a conversation about some contentious issue, they would probably readily say, there is always a possibility of being wrong. But especially after being in general practice or a specialist for years, the profound fundamental belief is likely to be, they always know best. The patient or student has trust in people who seem authoritative and their transference is in their obedience which might be unquestioning. (Also, counter transference, see below)

Personal Example I once raised serious questions about a presumptive medical diagnosis which had been handed to me (A Medical Misdiagnosis, see below). When I made an appointment at the local surgery, I expected normal treatment. I presented my concerns as logically as I could, only to find I was treated oddly. The doctor didn't bother to conceal her annoyance and called me a nuisance! I was astounded. I left, and worked on my situation, collecting data from medical records and seeking a second opinion. I got well with help from a consultant in a different county and eventually all concerned had to admit, I had been handed a false, presumptive diagnosis which had held up my recovery at the time. That surgery doctor was so used to working without being questioned, her transference made her very sure she was always correct and her instinctive reaction to my thought and questions was anger.

Counter Transference

Theory The unconscious process of counter transference which makes a person respond accordingly. In a psychological process, the responses and resultant actions which we seem to be required of us can be the ones we find ourselves engaging in even against our better judgment. We doubt ourselves and think the other person must be right.

People in general Faced with a person who has brought their particular way of being to the relationship or situation, a person might respond in a way that immediately picks up on what that first person has engendered, even responding in a way that is exactly what the first is looking for. It could be that, in counter transference, someone picks up on the absolute belief of another that they are not capable of making their own decisions. That more submissive person will then follow the wishes of the stronger character and it happens, essentially, because it's their habit.

Theoretical example It's not uncommon for a patient to recount the experience of entering a doctor's surgery knowing exactly what they wanted to describe and even knowing the outcome they hoped for, only to emerge feeling that something went wrong. They have accepted a fast diagnosis and a prescription but they are not quite sure it was the exact route they wanted. When doctors say you cannot get better or when they insist on treating your efforts to change your diet with lofty disdain, they are bringing along their old perceptions which they are resistant to altering. In your turn, you might get counter transference and think you must be in the wrong. You are not in the wrong. The typical family doctor is not often trained in psychology and won't realise he or she is just obeying unconscious habitual thought processes. In simple terms, the doctor finds it easier to make a set of assumptions which have been relied upon before. With courage, you can reject the self-doubt which then threatens to affect you.

Personal Example During the months when ME affected me, I was at risk of taking on board a certain perception inflicted on me, to the effect that I was odd. I was confounded by finding myself debilitated. I hated my condition and my vulnerable situation and it seemed a strange and unreal situation. My courage was there, however, submerged for a time by the genuine suffering and the highly sensitive feelings but not beaten away for good. I fought back against most of the cruel remarks and, when I was accused of being unusual, I found my voice and always insisted that ME could affect anyone. Part of me really knew I did *not* bring the illness on myself and, in fact, the more I got the blame, the more annoyed I felt and the surer I was, that I didn't deserve it.

So, I spotted my counter transference. I have explained that I could not contemplate letting a doctor tell me a second time that there was no cure and therefore I kept away from the surgery as much as I could.

Some sufferers may be luckier than I was and they may be able to find a sympathetic general practitioner or consultant. However, no matter how kind they seem, it's useful to be aware of the complicated processes of transference and counter transference and to look for absolute professionalism at all times.

Projection

Theory Someone who is adopting transference and is lofty and manipulative will then use projection to make the other person feel small. This perception, which may be unconscious, is designed to lift the burden of guilt from oneself.

It isn't me who is causing a problem! It's you!

Someone accuses another of the very set of thoughts and the same behaviour of which they, themselves are guilty. (If you apply this theory at those times when you have been absolutely confounded by the treatment you receive from another person, it really works!)

People in general Copying behaviour is useful example of projection. A tendency to be envious is a natural human instinct. For some, copying behaviour is intrinsic, and they clearly admire certain others, looking to have the same attributes or possessions, or do the same things. Celebrities gain such admiration and perhaps they look for it. In a personal sense, however, it can feel annoying regardless of the implied flattery.

As the subject of another's envy, perhaps one might mention this, but no matter how kindly the observation is phrased your copier may make accusations of selfishness and thinking that everything you do is so wonderful, no-one else can have the same things as you. They are defensive and this can turn to anger on their part. They do think you are enviable but, detesting this feeling in themselves and a sense of challenge which is a result of their own perception, they say, you believe yourself to be enviable. They might even say, *you* copy *them!*

Theoretical example Even a doctor might potentially accuse an ME patient of being obstructive in the course of their own recovery, but this is the result of his or her firm feeling that they have nothing more to offer. They won't research further on the patient's behalf. It's easier for them to say the patient is the one blocking the recovery, as opposed to admitting that they have chosen to come to a halt. In reality, *they* are weak, not the patient.

Family and friends who cannot bear to contemplate the effects of ME on the sufferer will tend to dismiss the whole problem from their consciousness. Your very existence in that condition presents them with their own inadequacies. They don't understand what's happening to you, and worse than that, they don't want to try to understand it.

You present a challenge to family and friends, who think you might hold them up in their lives. It's much easier to be around folk who don't seem to be a nuisance in any way, so they're sure it's you who must be considered unfair, and your behaviour must be untoward.

The truth is, they are not fair. They *say* you are handling your illness wrongly; you should do things differently and get better. What they mean is: don't even *be* ill. It bothers them because it seems to create a situation where something is required of them. Go forward and leave it behind you, they say, meaning you must leave it behind them, too. Get better magically and get better quickly! (If only you could.)

Personal Example When I was a child, a couple of youngsters in my life bullied me relentlessly. I had no way of avoiding them and it wasn't fair. Despite that, if I ever retaliated with angry words my parents were quick to reprove and blame me. I was slightly older than my tormentors and given to understand that I should be able to cope.

No-one enjoys being bullied and I didn't understand my enforced victimhood. Others were spiteful, but I was the one who was taken to task and reproved for reacting. I couldn't cope alone, and I used to hide in my room and cry.

When people felt inadequate to support the very ill person I became, they insisted it was I, who was inadequate, weak, unable to get myself together. I had to be in the wrong so they were not actually failing me.

Had a friend come to help me? No, falsely bright, she was determined she couldn't stay.

Had my mother called to offer help? No, she expressed exasperation.

Could someone come? My father said he couldn't; nor could my mother. He informed me that everyone feels tired sometimes.

In each of these scenarios, the person who showed me rejection and even hostility was applying their own inadequacies to me. I was supposed to be in the wrong, for being needy.

Do I forgive them, since it's possible they simply didn't know what to do? Forgiveness (fortunately) isn't essential to finding a way forward, in my experience.

If I was in that situation and if it was reversed, I would want to know what I could do to help. When a young mother has all her resources wiped out, doesn't she deserve help with the children, the chores and the shopping? Why not listen and try to be kind? Isn't it reasonable to support someone without judging them?

When someone seems to be accusing or reproachful towards you, and when this causes you frustration and feels very unfair, look for the projection. If it feels extraordinarily unfair then, undoubtedly, it is!

Psychological Blocks

In the quest for a route to good health it's worth considering anything and everything that might be getting in the way, and in this process it's important to examine your own mindset. As before, I would respectfully ask a reader to suspend disbelief and (of course) not take offence.

With an open mind, consider this:

What comprises your collection of basic ideas? They could be a set of beliefs which have been affected by other people, and which may be challenged.

Everyone says that ME is a mysterious illness. They debate whether or not its cause and manifestation constitute a disease process as such.

Everyone says, there's presently no cure.

Everyone is waiting for a new medicine to be invented. There is research ongoing, and many are determined that a pill will arrive.

You can make deliberate choices about these old fundamentals.

How about not caring how mysterious it's perceived to be, or (at least) setting that aside in your own mind? Not deliberating over how the phrase evolved, not interesting yourself in the fact that stating a mystery seems to let medical professionals off the hook in terms of addressing a cure?

Changing the phrase, *no cure* to read *route to recovery* opens up a possibility. Why not create an argument against being an ill person ongoing, even though there isn't a medical cure? Why not challenge and change the belief that there's no route to living as a well person?

One magical potion is envisaged? There isn't one yet, and all the argument seems increasingly muddled, even now, more than thirty years since I fell ill! Attempts to categorise different phases of the condition known as Myalgic Encephalomyelitis only muddy the waters, in my opinion. As I wrote near the start of this book, if the symptoms indicate ME, then it's ME. If they worsen, then management is failing or even harming the sufferer. There has to be another way forward.

With the emergence of vaccines, more than a couple in fact, during 2020 when the coronavirus pandemic began to cause widespread misery, it's not surprising that a certain belief exists and people trust in the scientists to bring out potions which seem almost magical. But the issue of long covid seems to be defying the medical profession and many of its symptoms are comparable to ME.

The Mindset

It's possible to pick up some thoughts and ideas which then feel definite and unalterable, but I firmly believe in lateral thinking. Your mindset is very important since, unless it is addressed, you will remain stuck.

Can you wait for a magic pill?

The thought of letting someone else step in and look after my two little boys was unwelcome and I dreaded such a thing. I was grateful for the kind assistance of my Nana for a time, but at least we were all in the same family home and I didn't have to let my sons go elsewhere. That fear was the best motivation I could have had, to throw myself at my research, my reading, the discoveries I could make in relation to vitamins and masked food allergy, and the new diet.

The sufferer has a train of thought that absolutely insists the medical profession must provide a cure. *If they have no medicine, then they need to invent one and cure my illness!* It is hard to let go of it, and that longing for the medical profession to take over this responsibility is entirely understandable.

For myself, I never went back to any doctor with issues relating to ME once I created my recovery plan via nutrition. The fact is, in relation to vitamins and what they do for us and what depletion causes, the work has already been done. It's deeply unfortunate that the general practitioner doesn't seem to have that knowledge in their armoury.

There's a feeling that ME sufferers dare not recover via diet for fear of letting the condition be minimised but I believe this has to be ignored, hard though it is. Even if the disbelievers think they gain grist to their mill, in fact, that isn't the case at all! You *were* ill, dreadfully so. If you get yourself feeling and looking fully well, this was a result of excellent management and truly, *you win!* No, you didn't get ill because of what you eat but yes, you can achieve wellness if you go the nutritional route.

Who cares what anyone thinks, if they are doubtful? You haven't lost face. You had a real condition but not a disease you couldn't beat. You triumphed!

Cognitive Dissonance

A mental or emotional struggle, often not at the surface of your thoughts but present in the back of the mind. It happens when something you need to do, or presently choose to do believing you are on the right track, conflicts with other beliefs you hold. Generally, it's something to avoid, being a stressful affect (in the Freudian sense) and one always feels more at ease after an important decision has been made and seems final. However, there are times when two issues cannot be fully resolved and differing feelings are inevitable.

For instance, I eat meat even though I am deeply compassionate towards animals. I was used to visiting farms as a child, but those experiences didn't turn me into someone who feels comfortable about eating meat, even though I gained an understanding of how responsible farmers approach and conduct their work. I don't eat meat every day, but the experience of being ill and recovering via nutritional approaches convinced me that I need to include it sometimes. And yet, I love and respect the animal world. The dilemma sometimes gives me nightmares. It's a problem of cognitive dissonance.

No Magic (The conflict for the person who contemplates abandoning the magic pill hopes.) To bring this issue into the frame I'm creating now, I need to explain that I completely understand how an ME sufferer might wish to keep their hopes for a miracle cure, hanging on to the idea that research will bring about a breakthrough and there will be a pill. Some people think finding a nutritional cure somehow negates the severity of the illness but it shouldn't and there are plenty **of** other ailments which may be improved with some kind of dietary approach.

If I let go, what have I said here? That I wasn't ill at all?

No; it's just a different way forward. If you can set aside that longing for medical help and your own resistance to what might happen if you try to change your diet (and pull all the strings I've discussed) and if you open your mind and let go of a feeling there is something to prove, you could make significant changes for yourself. The results could be great, with the conflict of beliefs thoroughly eclipsed by the outcome.

Going Forward (The conflict for the person who must change their perception of self.) Changes bring new challenges. It takes genuine courage to move forward into being fit and well, especially when you take the reins for yourself, and you may find the longing to get well is at odds with a train of thought. This affected me but I didn't emphasise it in No Medals because my sense of hesitation was a fleeting experience. I needed to transcend the feeling. However, it happened and perhaps it affects others.

When I thoroughly regained my energy, my days felt long because there were so many things I could do. I could let go of the ill person I had been. No doubt, I was still an ME "victim" but I had shed the symptoms and I no longer needed to feel or behave like a victim. I was thrilled, and yet there was a short time when I felt fearful. It was an odd contrast of emotions. There was vulnerability, almost as if I took my own safety net away. I dared to recover. A tricky memory; it's there but it slips away. We can develop a perception of ourselves which becomes habitual, and it isn't the same as being lazy or wanting to remain in an uncomfortable place. It can exist even when conscious thought says that place is unhappy, and freedom is the goal.

Slimmers who shed a lot of weight sometimes come up against an odd perception of themselves. Although they can look in the mirror or weigh themselves and know they lost weight, going forward their mind still tells them they are overweight!

As I grew stronger, there was briefly a sense (rather than a conscious thought) that I was worried about ways in which my life might alter. I had become accustomed, in a way, to the ill person I was. I felt challenged.

So, this is a tough thought process to revisit. What was at the root of this form of anxiety? Not the same as a panic attack, the feeling was hard to define. Did I want to stay in the role of a chronically ill patient?

No, my fears didn't mean I did wasn't longing to recover. However, I had become used to thinking of myself as being unwell. The situation had gone on for months and there were many things that were unhappy but unavoidable. Not being able to accept invitations … staying at home … living a quiet life … inevitably, avoiding challenges. For some, the months turn into years and a way of life is something one becomes used to. Like me perhaps, you have sadly become used to being treated a bit (or very) unkindly and a sense of victimhood isn't going to disappear overnight.

The more my mind fishes for the recollection of this confusing train of thought, the more it eludes me, and there are no conversations to recall. Who would have listened to me? So, the memory slips away, and there is no hardship or shame in moving away from that version of oneself, that ME victim who hoped and waited for medical treatment. I was ill and I needed and longed for some help, but I did it myself. A change happened and, in some ways, I whisked along quite fast. After being ill for more than two years, I recovered after a few false starts and more study and more attention to my diet, in about a month!

What is the obstacle in the way of confronting oneself as better? Perhaps its roots are in self-doubt and, in some ways, it feels baffling. Is it safer to stay at home, and be that ill individual? There is no shame in acknowledging this problem, and if it exists it doesn't detract from the patient's integrity. It's a change but there's no need to feel daunted; it's a good one. With courage, one can see there is no need to make a point to anyone else.

Getting well is the goal and it means everything to someone in the weakened, ill condition caused by Myalgic Encephalomyelitis. There is undoubtedly a need for courage, although it may not be so acute for ME victims who have been well-cared-for.

As soon as I stepped forward, fully, from the ill person I had contemplated being forced come to terms with, there was a renewed realisation. It was the fact that I really was on my own both physically and emotionally, not just during the bad time now passing but in the new phase. What would my life be like, from that point onwards? I had the physical recovery I craved but I was terribly hurt, emotionally. Could I forgive those who felt like bullies for that long, long time? Forgive the medical profession? Could I then, go out amongst people, and face a future where I might be challenged again?

As a matter of fact, I have never been able to place full trust in medical professionals ever since then. It's regrettable, but matters were not improved when I had an experience in later life which underlined my sense of an essential need to question treatment, always.

It takes courage to accept that most general practitioners cannot provide the ME patient with a safety net but I firmly believe it's a pity to waste time in waiting! Perhaps it's a big leap of faith in oneself but being brave enough not to need a "nice" doctor, at least in relation to the symptoms of ME, underlines the aim is simply to get well in a positive and logical way. That is, the doctor may be kind but if he or she has nothing to offer, then there's no real usefulness in trips to the surgery.

I would certainly have welcomed a kind attitude from someone who could support my mental recovery, but there was hardly anyone who cared enough to talk to me and my thoughts were still very much my own. I could never return to an agony aunt, knowing a different one could have the same perception as the woman who questioned my wish to be healthy and turn out to be just as damaging. I had developed an absolute hatred of seeing anyone purse their lips in response to something I said! Some people had been so unkind, I was still afraid of garnering more rude comments with implications about my character that would hurt for a lifetime.

I was once a child who often felt unhappy throughout the years of growing up, then as an adult that inner child stayed hurt. However, I made a deliberate choice. I went forward and kept links with my family. I still saw my parents, and chatted normally with them about everyday things. I didn't see any reason why my own children should be denied access to their grandparents as a result of the problems I had been handed.

I don't want to be disingenuous here. I recognise the huge emotional challenges that exist. I know the recovery can lead to a change in oneself along with many questions being presented. I maintain that they are questions which, in fact, one has no need to answer. People in general won't offer much of their time in any case.

So, how come you recovered? For the person who asks this, it could be quite a casual question. They might not expect anything much in reply, so be careful about your response and don't plunge into reflections and analysis unless all seems favourable and likely to lead to a reasonable conversation. They might knock you back but there is also a strong possibility they will not be interested enough to listen properly.

Of course, one can decide to create distance from the most toxic people, and on occasions when arguments and challenges are likely to be pointless, I do. I have mentioned above (Sugars) that, in confiding some of my experiences and thoughts, I encountered a woman who responded with sharp words to the effect that she thought she was listening to her body when she ate sugars. I made efforts to describe the way in which sugars can bring us down, making us tired but I knew she was entitled to her point of view and with counselling training I should respect that. However, I caught her in a sidelong glance with a roll of the eyes directed at someone else who was present, and I knew she was being contemptuous. She didn't mean well and with that realisation, I let her go.

Going On (The conflict for the person in recovery and socialising.) Once I had recovered, a terrific sense of excitement and achievement accompanied my feeling of good health. Sadly, I couldn't tell anyone! I felt different from other people because I had managed to pull myself through something big, but they only wished to make it small.

So, I chose to go forward in a life where I acted, mainly, as if nothing had happened. If I wanted to remain part of my wider family, a sort of pretence was the only framework I could construct for myself. No one would lend an ear, that was for sure! I hadn't really got much of an option if I wanted to stay a part of my family, not only for my sake but also for my children.

The sense of rising above something dreadful couldn't be dismissed, and yet no-one else cared! In a way, I lived in a void, somehow floating separately from others who would not acknowledge that something awful had happened. I had drawn on my resources of emotional strength, and found great courage, and yet I was considered odd. The illness had taken much of my freedom and my time away, but I had nowhere to take the thoughts.

The situation and, in fact, the ongoing sense of neglect made me feel angry. Often, I was in misery over the treatment I received, both during illness and as time went on, and I grieved, knowing I had lost much during the time I was so ill and was bullied. And yet I continued as if I had not.

When an individual tries to live with a sense of being at odds with their thoughts and actions, they may feel miserable. For many people, a moral conscience struggles to permit existence in that way, but when each of the conflicting arguments for certain actions is moral in itself, the difficulties are significant. I was angry and hurt, which made me sure it would have been justifiable for me to run away from the people who weren't kind or supportive. Yet, my little boys deserved to share time with my wider family, who were never going to harm them; on the contrary, I knew there were happy times ahead.

There were all the usual joyful milestones in their young lives. Jonathan left primary school to enter a middle school in Suffolk, while little Andy had a fourth birthday tea party which I'll never forget because of his laughter.

I was hurt but hopeful. I still felt part of my wider family and I had done nothing wrong. If it wasn't ideal, the fact was, I had become used to thinking nobody understood my plight (nor wanted to) and it's shocking to look back and realise I almost still thought I must be strange and different. With nobody in my life inclined to offer emotional comfort, who was going to help me get the strength to look objectively at everything? I was still quite young and I couldn't have reviewed the onslaught of illness plus insults in a dispassionate or objective way.

Life went on; there were events where my compassion was called upon and I couldn't ignore my natural instincts. If someone who was linked to me and part of my wider family became ill, I was kind. However, often people did return to me, looking for contact as if nothing had happened, and although I responded I suffered from confusion sometimes. It was common for familiar people to act as if they hadn't known about my diagnosis, or (more correctly) as if, knowing, they didn't care and yet still wanted to communicate their own troubles!

On form and feeling well, I can be animated, even funny, and that became a version of myself which I saw was acceptable again, to many.

A handful of friends hadn't been aware of my long illness and deserved no reproach, simply having thought we had temporarily lost touch in the way people sometimes do. Two old friends, unconnected with one another, had other acquaintances who suffered from ME. Based on what they understood of their friends' lives, they told me they knew my situation was hard *but you just have to pace yourself* or *it's nothing to do with food ...*

Hindsight brings many different reflections. Trying to put a bad time behind you often results in depression or anxiety but I wasn't depressed. I was so thrilled to feel well. Nevertheless, there was an effect in that I tended to suffer from outbursts of temper which were not consistent with my natural good humour. It was years before I understood that this was the result of trying to fit in with family gatherings without being able to mention my illness and everything that went with it. I still felt angry, of course I did, and sometimes I would sink into memories provoked by a thoughtless remark, or a radio or television feature about ME.

Mourning

I found comfort in small ways during the long months of illness. I could enjoy the endearing behaviour of my children, and in warm weather I could sit outside the house on my better days and make the most of the sunshine. I had to live very quietly. Essentially, I lost between two and three years of a full, active life. My situation seemed unreal at times and I grieved over it. How would those times have been different, had I not fallen ill after my second child was born?

I would have been more typically active, taking the boys swimming each week, playing with them instead of weakly watching while they made their own fun. We could have set off for the beach, sometimes. I would have ridden the little mare I was offered on loan. I could have attended the wedding of an old friend, instead of being utterly confounded by any thoughts of the many, normally joyful aspects of being a wedding guest. How would I dress myself smartly, or shop for a gift for the bridal couple, or tolerate the drive to the wedding venue? I couldn't, and I had to regretfully decline the invitation.

We must go forward after a shock and I did. I've discussed transcending fear, but it's hardly surprising that I was almost overwhelmed by sorrow even after I could walk again. Of course, I was saddened. How complex it was, considering the illness itself was nightmarish and so were others' responses. I didn't realise I was going through a grieving process which was entirely justifiable.

In a very human response, it became very hard to feel pity for family members, almost no matter what their ailments were! Few people escape an occasional cold virus or a bout of influenza. I felt renewed shock, any time I was asked to sympathise with someone who had formerly rejected me and yet now wanted to confide. Also, I developed an almost obsessional dislike of asking for help, even when it might have been forthcoming.

Did I go back, really, to the person I was before? I never weighed up that issue in the first few years after my recovery, even though I was often conscious of feeling awkward or annoyed by comments which showed family members were ignoring my experience. In some ways, there was devastation of the person I was before. There were ongoing effects on my character and they included confusion, anger, hurt, resentment and a sense of low self-worth. Most shocking of all, I retained a feeling that life is all about a lonely struggle and on some level, not even particularly unconscious, I doubted I deserved to be peaceful and happy. I had learned the lesson I developed and thoroughly taught myself. ME symptoms aren't to be battled but understood and dealt with. However, I felt as if life itself was intrinsically hard for me.

* * *

When I felt strong enough to visit a hairdresser, it was a real milestone in my recovery. I made an appointment, planned a hairstyle, and decided to take my small son along, too. The tiny salon in Bury St Edmunds was warm, perfumed and cosy. There was a hum of conversation all around us and Andrew happily sat on my lap, holding a storybook and chatting. Before long, leaning on me, he was overcome by the soporific atmosphere and fell asleep.

The hairdresser had pinned up her own hair into a beautiful blonde swirl. She made the usual small talk, while she combed and snipped my hair into a bobbed style. Had I been away on holiday lately?

No, I said. I had been very unwell, and was now recovering. I was very much looking forward to arranging some kind of holiday as soon as I felt strong enough to travel. Even short distances were still a challenge ... but my words petered out. My thoughts were numerous and I felt challenged by their complexity. There were linked problems, including the mental strain of planning a holiday. Mainly, I was worried about my stamina on any journey, regardless of my choice of transport. The hairdresser picked up on the first point.

"You were ill?"

I could see her reflection in the mirror, and she was looking away to our right, watching a colleague who was greeting another client. Absently, she ran a comb through a strand of my hair several times. I said, I had a virus. It was a conscious choice to avoid trying to describe what had been happening to me. Simply, I went on. "Yes, I was really ill. I'm alright now." There was a pause. Andy snoozed on, and my mind wandered back to my days of illness. "I never really knew it was possible to suffer so much in your own home ..." I said, thoughtfully.

The hairdresser was ready to concentrate again on the work in hand. Stooping, she frowned down at the hair strand as she expertly snipped. "Suffer?" She repeated the word without emphasis.

I dragged my thoughts back to the present and changed the subject. It was one of the first times, post illness, that I saw a further discussion of my experience wasn't necessary, or even wise. The whole thing was outside this young woman's frame of reference, kind though she was. Her world was all about clients, hairstyles and treatments, and keeping an eye on her younger trainees.

My Beliefs

In conversation with a small group of women, the subject of stress-related illness arose and my companions were emphatic. Migraine headaches, they declared, were the direct result of feeling stressed.

It's an interesting issue. I tended to suffer from migraine when I was a young woman, and it was a nuisance. As a personal assistant in a busy solicitor's office, suddenly being unable to see properly was a warning sign which also meant I was in for a nasty headache within the hour. It was a highly charged environment sometimes, where typists had to hammer out legal documents quickly and correctly. However, I had learned something and it was at least as important to me as the element of emotional pressure, so I volunteered it.

"Look out for eating sugars and sour food at the same meal!"

I described a painful experience, when I swiftly developed a migraine attack after eating a grapefruit followed by a bar of dark chocolate. The headache was excruciating and I was very sick, too. (As for this odd way of eating, in my defence I was only aged about twenty!)

But food combinations seem unimportant to many people, and while I would be happy to discuss the fact that they may firmly believe they are not affected, still, I was disappointed on that occasion, when my companions felt sure I was talking rubbish. I was an

ME survivor, but I had no *clout!* Naturally, they each had a perspective on the issue, but then they joined together in assuring me that migraines are due to stress, and stress alone. In conversation, this kind of argument does create some disappointment for me, as well as a feeling of frustration because I know that open-mindedness can lead to great things.

When people form a group, often they will copy the person who feels the most likely to lead them and their comments and behaviour can be blinkered. It turned out that I was the rejected individual on that occasion. My mild observation that becoming hungry can be a factor in developing a migraine was also unpopular and comments were even unpleasantly hostile, especially when I went on to say that drinking alcohol can affect a susceptible person!

The main thing for me, was my ability to manage my health and linked conditions. While my companions preferred to decide that migraine is some kind of mystery and singularly a stress response; clearly, I could easily afford to make up my own mind and continue in my own way.

* * *

With a fascination with good health which has lasted, I have sometimes joined online courses, looking at the management of different illnesses where conditions respond to a change of diet and have the potential to change with immaculate attention to good nutrition. When I studied aspects of diabetes, I was one of the older participants who could all remember the condition being referred to as *sugar diabetes* by adults around us, when we were young.

I read about people who had managed pre-diabetes conditions via their diet and inevitably I wrote enthusiastically about my huge efforts to get over ME. I described something of what I did and what happened, putting my posts on a forum for discussion with other learners. Someone posted a lofty reply.

"Ah. If only it were that simple, Lisette!"

It's a fact that altering and fully overhauling your diet is far from simple. *Good nutrition* might be a phrase easily said or written, but the study of vitamins and what they can do for you, and the ailments that can result from depletion, can be as complicated as you want to make it. There is so much to learn. As for having the courage to learn while you are ill and debilitated, to open your mind to theories such as masked food allergy, to try it for yourself, and to set aside some of the foods you thought of as comforting: it's all far from simple.

Certain foods create a sense of comfort which may be remembered from our childhood, when tastes, habits and associated feelings form. Foods that are part of our culture pass on through generations from our parents. To address a complete change in eating habits, one needs courage, an open mind and self-belief. It's important to find a way to view the body and system as the flesh and blood being it is, and understand that thoughts and emotions will have to be guided away from the old habits. When you read these books, let ideas flow and try not to put mental blocks in the way of developing a personal plan which could help in the quest for strength and wellness.

Where another condition exists along with all the symptoms of ME, then there's no question at all about the advisability of seeking advice and support from a doctor. However, it would be saddening if a medical professional who is asked to help at such a time expresses doubt which could affect a patient's resolve. For myself, unless such comments raise genuine, specific problems which are directly prohibitive of improved nutrition, then I would want a second opinion.

In terms of making comparisons with other people, it can be interesting and even useful to share experiences with another sufferer but it's essential to evolve a way that suits you personally. Gather positive ideas from others but don't labour over the negative remarks. It's time to put yourself first.

All too often, as soon as I mention nutrition, a sufferer will say something careless. *Oh, I don't care what I eat!* They can't be bothered to think about changing their diet. Instead of the key to the future, they think the idea is nothing but a nuisance. Sometimes, the ME sufferer is already so uncomfortable and unwell, they're sure they may as well have whatever they want.

One lady who had been ill for years was said to be immediately dismissive when her friend told her about my recovery. "I just have chocolate for breakfast …"

A well person can get away with chocolate for breakfast. An ill person needs to do much better than that. In the field of nutrition and vitamins and how they affect us, a world of knowledge can be found, and offers a wonderful opportunity to begin creating a recovery from ME. Food *does* make a difference.

So, is it hard or easy to adopt a nutritional approach and seek a cure for the affliction and its multitude of symptoms? Is it akin to rocket science, or not? Learning about the various vitamins, understanding masked food allergy, and importantly gaining a good picture of the workings of your own bodily system, *and* keeping at it even when you feel unwell and discouraged? Letting go of some foods which you have thought of as comforting, perhaps since childhood. These things are definitely all hard.

It's common to present a picture of a typical ME sufferer with emphasis on all the poorly outward signs of the condition. A photograph shows the person lying in bed, looking wan, looking unhappy and exhausted. Those of us who have gone through that miserable time will identify with this depiction, but it's unfortunate that many will reject it. It doesn't help, actually, to draw others in and it cannot create interest in the condition, nor is it likely to gain sympathy.

Oh, but it's a real condition!

Offended, many sufferers may insist that these pictures are essential. Why should other people ignore the way we sometimes look, or turn away from the illness that seems to plague us? This is understandable, and so is a certain determination to keep with the typical attitudes but a change in style could bring benefits.

I don't think emphasising the dreadful symptoms, or photographing people with pale, tired faces will help to convince anyone who prefers to doubt us. Really, the ME victim is sunk in terms of respect from others who know nothing about the illness, by the fact that the medical professionals have nothing much to offer. Perhaps your personal story emerges in the future, and perhaps respect will follow; but meanwhile you just have to be very brave. It's so difficult to describe the way you feel when you know people are disinterested or even wary.

* * *

It's my belief that the collection of symptoms which can be identified under the heading of Myalgic Encephalomyelitis reflect a profound, catastrophic depletion in the essential vitamins. This can occur after a period of illness which may be viral, but there are other ways in which a person may be reduced to a state of exhaustion overall. The body produces a range of symptoms to alert the system to this and in identifying the symptoms collectively as one enemy, in fact, I think the patient is misguided.

It's important to look at what each symptom indicates, and tackle that vitamin deficiency. To this statement, I would add the issue of masked food allergies which are specific to each sufferer. They don't seem to be harmful to everyone, certainly not to people who are generally well, but attention to this theory and application during illness can be invaluable.

No, there isn't a medicine to cure the symptoms overall.

Yes, the answer is there and it lies in science. It's the science of how the human body works.

* * *

The way forward lies with good nutrition, and also good management which must never result in extra exhaustion. An ME sufferer cannot expect a great result if they are forced to be physically or mentally active. In No Medals, I wrote about my *collapsed puppet* and my *beautiful racehorse* theories. These are positive ideas, and they do work well.

I'm incredulous when I read dismissive comments from very experienced, erudite medical people. *We simply haven't the knowledge to treat these things.* They have! Look at the vitamins, the ailments that come from depletion of those essential elements. In my little book (The Vitamins Explained Simply) I found that precious statement about needing more if you are ill.

It's important to avoid repetitive eating of any type of food, and also not to get addicted to any type of drink. Once you feel better, adopt moderation in all things and the wonderful reward for all the hard work on your diet can be a sense of being truly refreshed.

If you work on your diet with a view to avoiding repetitive eating, you might find yourself taking something out that does presently cause problems but also is generally a food that offers benefits. So, for instance, perhaps eggs need to be left alone for a week or so while you shake up your meals and make them different, but other sources of protein will need to be found as a substitute. Of course, the assistance of a nutritionist or dietician could be helpful.

* * *

There is no need to feel hungry and it's not indicated at all, but it's a good idea to substitute sweet treats such as chocolate bars with foods that offer benefits. Choose fresh fruit, or brown bread, toasted perhaps, and spread with honey or peanut butter. Calories need to be worth more than just a moment's comfort.

Similarly, savoury snacks like crisps are not going to help you feel well but something simple like hot noodles may satisfy a persistent appetite in a healthy way, or begin to retrain an appetite that's weak.

I am well aware that this is very difficult for anyone who has an eating disorder. In that connection, of course, the mental health issues surrounding anorexia nervosa or bulimia, and the effects they have on the sufferer's physical condition, are not part of my personal experience and therefore my understanding of them isn't for me to convey in this book.

* * *

Someone who struggles with overweight may feel certain they don't actually overeat. That's a simple statement, but it can be maddening to a person who thinks for sure, it's true of them. They want to believe their intake is satisfactory, and so they convince themselves it's true.

The multitude of problems with overweight include a complicated set of issues caused by hormones (such as ghrelin), which are linked with the brain and gut, and which stimulate appetite.

There's homeostasis, which is the body's way of returning to a satisfactory state as soon as possible after a dietary change, and which explains why many weight loss diets fail in the long run as the system adjusts, and learns to maintain a certain weight using fewer calories.

Then, there are issues such as comfort eating. It's especially significant in someone who tends to turn to the foods they enjoyed as a child, whether that's because the memories are happy or because the memories of those times were harmed in some way by the behaviour of someone. With different causes, the result is that food feels comforting.

There are issues such as failing to be active, not using up calories because of limited exercise, and for some people, that is beyond their control when they are not well or disabled. So, it's not simple.

Nevertheless, I would draw a respectful comparison between a person who does overeat, and anyone who needs to adjust their diet for any other reason. (For example, pre-diabetes is said to be possible to alter via a nutritional approach.) The usefulness of keeping a food diary can't be overstated, and while it might be discarded at a later date, during a period of recovery it's really worthwhile. An account of dietary intake every day helps the overweight person to keep calories low, and for anyone tracing food and drinks which are best eliminated from their diet for the time being, a written record supports that effort.

* * *

Food or drinks containing caffeine are best avoided while the effort to recover from ME is ongoing. Every so often, invisible researchers turn out to be really sure that caffeine is good for you. I have heard this debated by a doctor on a television programme, who acknowledged that coffee gives some people a nervous, jittery effect or even a headache, and yet still insisted the research is valid. When I gradually weaned myself off caffeine (in tea, coffee and chocolate) I was uncomfortable for a few days and I had withdrawal headaches, but I achieved a feeling of freshness.

I sacrificed the lift of a small hit of caffeine and freed myself of the craving, and then this meant that I didn't have those lows which can come when the body starts to demand a new hit of caffeine again. It was a relatively small thing to do for myself, albeit quite difficult, but it had a great outcome.

Some people swap caffeinated tea and coffee for the decaffeinated kind. I didn't, preferring herbal teas and freedom from the addiction, but it's one way to avoid feeling deprived of something you enjoy.

MASKED FOOD ALLERGY (SPECIFIC ALLERGIC ADAPTATION)

Don't shoot the messenger!

The bearer of unwelcome or awkward news isn't at fault and the message could have its value. This theory is tricky, but it's clever. I tried it out in a careful way, and found I could make it work for me and I'm glad it never crossed my mind to dismiss it out-of-hand. It was a game changer. I can't believe it's thought contentious or unlikely to be useful! Those old designations are so unfortunate! *ME is a mystery ... masked food allergy is contentious.* Such habitual descriptions need to be thrown out and minds need to be opened.

What use is there, in turning away without investigating something, saying *I've heard of that and it's said to be rubbish*? Why not read about the theory and the case studies, considering each detail very carefully? Especially where any of the cases seem to have *any form of* relevance to your own experience. Then, why not try it?

There are aspects of the application of the theory which need working on in order to produce the best outcome for the patient. In an ideal world, doctors would learn about it and apply it too. I can try to explain how I managed to use it to my absolute advantage.

I had regained a considerable amount of energy and wellbeing after a few weeks on my plan, building better foods into my daily consumption, including fruits and vegetables, and taking care over carbohydrates and proteins ... and so on. I could go outside into sunlight, enjoy it and know I was receiving Vitamin D at the same time. I was beginning to remember what it was like to feel well. Inevitably, I was confounded when I began to slip back into a state of discomfort and sleepiness. My faith in nutritional cures had been growing, and I would not give in. I felt sure there must be some reason to pinpoint and I was equally sure it would relate to my food.

I delved back into my pile of books and found one which I had set aside to begin with. Not All in the Mind by Dr Richard Mackarness looked interesting, and the only reason I hadn't turned to it before was the revelations about vitamins and their deficiency results had seemed enough.

I read this book, was drawn in and became fascinated by the case studies. None were a perfect match for my situation and they were surprisingly varied, but they seemed to hold very big clues nonetheless. The messages about recovery were there; they seemed promising, and I resolved to try the system. I would try the avoidance of repetitive eating. For my part, I quickly found that once I had identified repetitive eating and removed a food from my diet for four days, gone through headaches and malaise on about the second and third days and felt better afterwards, then I could reintroduce a small quantity of the same food. I didn't have to write it off forever. There isn't anything wrong with that, at all! Do I care about how this actually worked? Not a bit!

I realised I was eating the same breakfast every day: typically, porridge. I had introduced porridge in my diet to make sure I ate a sustaining breakfast and it's a great food in itself, but I had certainly formed a habit of eating it often. I altered my habits at breakfast time and cut out oatmeal for three days then reintroduced it, being careful to eat something different on alternative days.

This sounds simple: *avoid repetitive eating of any type of food.* Yet, it's complicated as soon as you wonder: *why on earth is this so important?* I didn't care about the reason why! I could walk without shaking and I felt so refreshed.

When I addressed my repetitive eating, for three days in a row I substituted a completely different breakfast. Sometimes, I would make poached egg on toast; others, I ate fresh seed bread and honey, and occasionally I had yoghurt. I don't think yoghurt alone is sustaining enough for an ME sufferer and I always added some fruit. Days on, when I ate a small amount of porridge again, I was fine, but I made sure I didn't start to repeat it daily. (I never have!)

Some people who wouldn't consider themselves unwell, nevertheless will confess to feeling sleepy after eating sugars. This is a mild acknowledgement of how food can affect us, and there is no reason why one should not develop that type of thought and analysis.

Some experiences on this route can be quite dramatic. I remember the moment I drank lemonade thinking it would be a refreshing alternative to alcohol, only to find I felt horrible! I had achieved a certain level of improved wellness by then; I was drinking more water, making sure to have breakfast and other important meals, but I hadn't yet tried the masked food allergy system. I wasn't drinking wine. Feeling as if I had made a wise choice, I poured a glass of lemonade. When I drank it and then it obviously gave me a headache, I remember exclaiming aloud! "Oh! It must be *all* sugars!"

I was very sensitive at that point, and realising sugar was a problem really was a lightbulb moment.

It wouldn't be completely honest to move on from this chapter without mentioning that the headaches and malaise during a period of withdrawal from a type of food may be quite unpleasant. For me, headaches were persistent during the first couple of days and there was a feeling of tension. A few times, I had restless sleep, even nightmares, and up until the fourth day minus the food I was eliminating, I was rather flat in my mood. But after those difficult days, I felt better.

At last, my recovery seemed certain. I had suffered many ups and downs, and after all it was a process of trial and error, deliberately experimenting and looking for answers. In the end, I felt truly refreshed. In the mornings, waking, I had the same feeling as a cool shower or light summer rain on the face, or a swim in the sea which invigorates the mind and body. It was wonderful!

University Centre: A Person-Centred Counselling Course

In a classroom setting, I was a mature student when a tutor who was aware of my writing showed a real interest in No Medals for ME. He chatted to me privately and explained that he thought my book was truly reflective of the person-centred model in counselling. He promised me an opportunity to present it to a group of trainee counsellors. I was pleased, and wrote a presentation plan, considered my time frame and selected the main points I would emphasise. I had experience of doing the same at Essex Authors' Day.

The tutor's interest in me and my work didn't come to anything and I found at a later date there was resentment from his superior. It was something to do with my prior learning and my ability to question our course presentations. (It's another story!) In hopes, I went ahead and prepared my presentation with careful attention to all the details that mattered to me, but the head of department made things difficult and I never presented the book to my classmates. However, one afternoon there was a discussion of the overall concept of illness which seems to arise from emotional upset. Someone referred to ME and I found an opportunity to talk.

I explained a few things, speaking without the benefit of my notes but from the heart. It's physical, I said, but I acknowledged the fact that victims often become very sensitive.

I thought the group was listening. Around twenty classmates

included mature students like myself, and an equal number of younger people in their very early twenties. They seemed to be paying attention but, as things turned out, no-one was particularly interested. I finished speaking and the tutor (a very young woman) made a comment.

"As Lisette has mentioned, this kind of thing is mainly linked with mental illness!"

What a disappointment! Her comment didn't reflect my points; instead, it showed she *hadn't* listened properly. Wordless then, I sat on at my table and chose not to challenge her. We were in a classroom, after all. My role was that of student at that time, so a furious argument would have been inappropriate and probably would only have wrecked my case!

Inevitably, the classmates took their cue from their tutor, and conversation moved into discussions about anxiety and stress. No-one seemed to spot that a person who had survived ME could be more likely to enlighten them about the condition, compared with a young woman whose learning was mainly the skimmed surface of a handful of theories.

This was a course which I undertook in a university centre, where I attended with hopes of thorough enjoyment of erudite studies but was sadly disappointed. I found the presentations compared unfavourably with my prior learning and personal experience. They were often painfully inadequate, the study material we were offered was generally out-of-date, and tutors had not trained further than the most basic of person-centred theories and couldn't conceal the fact they had scant teacher training. They were proud of their achievements, but it was apparent that their achievements weren't many.

One can take useful messages from experiences in any learning centre, but I was surprised and shocked when I found the level of education didn't match other studies which I had undertaken in a different university, and even in adult community education. Trainees were permitted to move on from the role play which was included during the first few months, and they could begin counselling real clients after just one academic year. As the months rolled on and the process commenced there was confusion for many, who went headlong into a situation they were not equipped to handle.

A fully trained, well-educated counsellor can do a wonderful job, but someone who undertook just a couple of years to gain a diploma may not have all the deep knowledge of aspects of psychology which they need. Enthusiasm and a certificate to prove they produced a series of essays (which they may have made several attempts to pass), bears little comparison with extensive life experience and it's not satisfactory minus brilliant tuition in surrounding subjects. It's unfortunate that some who believe themselves to be well able to support distressed people, simply aren't good enough. They are likely to imagine their hypotheses are of equal value to well-educated awareness and, in my experience, they can become self-important (even though it's the last thing they are supposed to do), sometimes even using inappropriate challenges which risk harming the peace of mind of the client.

During a time when symptoms of ME are ongoing, a person-centred counsellor might be great, as long as they are respectful. It goes without saying, too, that the patient needs to be in a condition where they are able to talk without suffering extra debilitation. The counselling process will not be worthwhile, however, if the therapist tries out their own ideas in a speculative way (as opposed to an informed way). Unfortunately, those who achieved nothing more than a diploma over two years do tend to imagine their guesswork is the same as learned understanding. Worst of all, could be the ones who think that, if they support your mental health, you'll get better from ME.

With counselling training, I know the enormous value of therapy when it's appropriate, and I have comprehensively studied the person-centred model as well as psychodynamic theories. I spent some time working through courses in aspects of psychology, including forensic and observational approaches. The ME patient is going through a hellish experience, and that's true even if they are being treated kindly. The gentlest, most compassionate form of person-centred counselling might have its place eventually but while someone is so weak that they can barely talk, it's not the right thing to do. Sometimes, following a counselling session, the mind will race. It's best to stay as calm and quiet as possible during acutely painful illness, and seek counselling after the worst is over. (Hopefully, once a nutritional plan has helped to bring about a good change!) It's not time to begin therapy while the sufferer is hardly able to pick up a toothbrush and brush their teeth.

Going forward, in making choices about the very best type of therapy I would insist that cognitive behavioural therapy (CBT) isn't a good idea. There must be no forcing, physically. Behavioural changes may follow regained wellbeing; otherwise, the counselling could do more harm than good. Also, I'd say (for the time being) avoid psychotherapy. The ME patient doesn't need to be psycho-analysed; not while they are physically ill.

In No Medals, I explained that I knew a psychologist might want to suggest I was bringing further illness upon myself because I knew as I fell asleep that I would not wake up cured. They would be wrong, and the illness was nothing to do with my mental strength.

HATTIE

Years ago, except for the false tag of "Yuppie Flu", there weren't the same definitions which seem to have emerged with regard to differing types of ME. (Or, if they had begun to be considered, they weren't highlighted in articles I read.)

I have explained that, when I refer to the condition I had as a young woman, I absolutely intend to refer to Myalgic Encephalomyelitis. Not even CFS, although I recognise there could be significant comparisons with my experiences in every sense.

Additionally, I cannot buy into the more recent detailed lists which I have seen, where ME is split into types according to severity. Certainly, there are those who experience the early stages differently from the more intense debilitation and suffering that can come later (not for everyone, but that does depend on how carefully the illness is managed) but if it's ME, I'd say, it has the potential to go from bad to worse and still be the same condition overall. It also has the potential to ease.

However, while I maintain this belief, I acknowledge the reflections that could arise for the reader when I describe my friend, Hattie; and the fact that I almost look as if I turn my own perception on its head! True histories of other sufferers, or in this case, someone who might have been a sufferer, can bring many reflections and sometimes enlightenment to a certain extent.

I was introduced to Hattie by a kind person who came to talk to me following a sad bereavement in 2002. For this book, I'll refer to her as Mrs G. She spent some time listening to my reflections, and one day, they included the subject of ME and my struggle then, and the ways in which I found some similarities in bereavement. People not knowing what to say, or (worse) saying appalling things, figured large.

Mrs G had a friend whose daughter, aged about thirty, never seemed to feel well. Putting Hattie and myself in touch with one another was a stroke of genius. I was suffering, lost in time in a way, but needing to get through a dreadful period in my life. I was trying to be a good mother to my remaining children but I needed to regain my self-esteem. Hattie lived a lonely life in a countrified place, with her mother but without neighbours, and she was limited by her set of health issues. Respectfully, I asked what they were, inasmuch as I was allowed to know.

"She walks with difficulty, and sometimes feels she can't walk at all. She bumps into the furniture all the time! She's funny, and often laughs at herself, but you almost feel she could get lost in her own home. She seems to take information on board, but then she can't remember it later. Her mother and sister are sure that she wouldn't be able to live alone.

"Yet, some things about her would make you think she was very able: even gifted! She is highly intelligent, loves books and films, takes an interest in the world ... and she loves to talk."

So, armed with a scribbled map, one afternoon I set off in my car to visit Hattie, after our mutual friend made the arrangements for us.

Hattie came to meet me when I drew up before a wide gate. She was leaning on a stick but needed no strength to open the gate, which easily swung open once unlatched. I had to slip through a narrow space, to make sure her two dogs couldn't run away.

"Would they ...?" I asked.

"It's been known," Hattie said, with a grin. "Come on!"

We walked over a springy, mown lawn, ducking our heads beneath the low branches of apple trees, and passing rockeries and flowerbeds. There were rose bushes where an older lady, Hattie's mother was busy with secateurs. She waved to me in a brief acknowledgement.

I was charmed by Hattie's home. The cottage was tiny, and inside it was beamed and full of typical countrified things: flower print armchairs, an open fire, a Welsh dresser made of dark wood (stained oak, perhaps). Framed photographs were everywhere, hanging on walls and placed on low tables, and pictures of beloved dogs had been given at least equal pride of place compared with those of humans. The book case was full and included books written by Hattie's father, now deceased. She told me he was an erudite man. It was a peaceful, country atmosphere. Completing the picture and the genuine enjoyment I had in visiting, were the two wagging spaniels.

Hattie and I became friends very quickly. I recognised her lively interest in the world and I really liked the way I could confidently chat to her about my history of education, which had been hidden from others in terms of conversation for many years. Hattie respected educated people. I had long felt that I was educated for something I never really achieved, and some of my grammar school friends had gone on to be teachers, solicitors, or people with enormous responsibility in the media. Now, the way I spoke and the things I knew were appreciated, and Hattie saw no difference between myself and the high achievers I described. I didn't mention ME at first, finding my way, wanting to be friendly without looking intrusive.

One afternoon, when the fire blazed in the hearth and the dogs slept on the rug near our feet, Hattie brought me a cup of tea, then returned to the kitchen to pour a glass of cola for herself. When she returned, we sat quietly for a moment or two. It was an effort for

Hattie to make tea, and I knew that. She had asked what I normally like to drink, and I had mentioned herbal teas but I enjoyed a cup of ordinary tea, although I never brewed it for long. After a few minutes, tentatively I asked about her love of cola.

"Go and look in the larder!" she said, with a smile. I obeyed, and found ten or more bottles on the stone floor, and they were full of cola, orange fizzy, and other types of lemonade. *Oh!* She was addicted to those drinks, I realised. I went to join her again and I was smiling too. When I expressed my thoughts, Hattie agreed: yes, she was addicted to soft drinks.

By this time, I felt I could ask her a question. Had she ever had a diagnosis for the collection of ailments that affected her? Her difficulties in walking, the sense of weakness, and so on? The tendency to have good days and bad? The chilly feeling which could persist even on a sunny day, and her memory problems? Could these things all be a result of having ME?"

Hattie knew all about it and I didn't have to explain further, but when she responded, somehow, she killed the subject. "The doctor says, it's not ME."

What did she think about that? I wondered, but she had spoken with an air of finality. The question felt like a step too far, so I kept it to myself and I didn't press her to try to elaborate. As time went on, we had more conversations and Hattie showed she was not particularly reluctant to discuss her condition but she simply didn't know what caused it. On one occasion, I contemplated seeing a doctor or consultant for some ailment (now forgotten), and she had a curt retort accompanied by her characteristic, wide grin. *"They don't know anything!"*

Every year at Christmas time, she sent me a card, just a flimsy one selected from a box of mixed designs. It usually bore a traditional depiction of the Nativity scene. Inside, awkwardly written, were the words: *love from Hattie*. Once, I bought a pair of fluffy socks and wrapped them up as a small gift for her, and she was very pleased. She felt cold all the time, and wore a knitted hat every day.

Her life went on in the same way for a few years, and I visited quite often, and she seemed to enjoy listening to me talk about my family and my interests. When I began to train as a counsellor, she was warmly supportive. The active life I led was of genuine interest to Hattie, and she was a true friend who showed no envy or malice, ever. When I visited her on a chilly day wearing a new coat, she said, generously, that I looked fantastic!

Then Hattie's mother passed away. Supported for a few weeks by a relative who went to stay with her in the cottage, Hattie coped at first but her disabilities included dyspraxia; she was uncoordinated in her movements and, for this reason and others, she was deemed vulnerable. Unable to be left, safely, on her own, she had to go into a type of sheltered accommodation. I visited her during those early weeks after her sad loss, and I wondered how badly she might be affected by this big change to her life. With the death of her mother, there were other losses too, including her beautiful home and her dear dogs.

Hattie was stoic, and in fact her courage was admirable. She wasn't inclined to talk about her mother, but she showed me photographs of the dogs and said, confidently, they had been given to kind new owners. This must have given her comfort, and she didn't seem to find the parting too painful. She would see them again, she told me. As for ourselves and our friendship, we would keep in touch with one another.

My visits to the pretty cottage were over but I was invited to the new flat where Hattie was safe and comfortable. All over the walls, on a level with her eyeline, there were notes stuck there with tape and they were reminders and *to do* lists. She laughed at herself.

"I forget to look at them!"

By this time, I was quite well aware that if I pressed her to get extra help to review her health, Hattie could become irritable and I learned not to do it. Then, things got sad because she stopped eating. She just stopped. Once again, she seemed slightly outside of any typical diagnostic framework. Was she suffering from anorexia nervosa? No, her mental state didn't seem that complicated. Nor bulimia. She was at peace with herself and quite liked life; she simply stopped eating and absolutely didn't want to. For about a year and a half, incredibly, I knew the medical profession kept her alive with a feeding tube at night, while she slept.

Was that horrible? I asked. Wouldn't it be more comfortable and nicer, to have a few little meals in the daytime? No, that comment was unwelcome and good tempered, funny Hattie was obviously about to get irritated about it, if I went on! She mentioned in a factual way that her canula was a nuisance, but that was all she would say about it. She liked to call me on the telephone in the evenings, and the things she told me seemed to reflect a fairly contented life. She had a friend with similar disabilities but, leaning on their sticks, they could walk a short distance to the nearest bus stop and they like to catch a bus to Wivenhoe, where they watched the boats in the harbour. She was full of humour, living her life as well as she could, and when she described him, it seemed to me that her friend may have been a boyfriend.

I had changed my own circumstances and my days were very full. One evening, I realised I had no mental picture of Hattie's surroundings any more. She was living in a new flat, more protected as she had to be since the refusal to eat began, and being visited regularly by a nurse. I was unsure where the building was.

"I need to come and see you again!" I told her.

Hattie agreed but said she thought everything was alright. She liked talking on the telephone and she reassured me, saying I would see her soon. She was given sleeping medicine with her night-time liquid diet though, and once or twice she began to snore before we ended the conversation. She was asleep!

Then her calls stopped. I became aware of it after a few weeks and, with a sinking heart, I rang the familiar number and got a disconnected tone. The use of the flats had altered; I couldn't trace Hattie, and circumstances were against my efforts. I had no right to investigate via the hospital because I was not a relative. The kind lady who introduced us in the first place had moved away to a different county, and although I found her new address after some weeks of trying, when I contacted her, it was only to find she had lost touch with Hattie's mother and, with the passing of that lady, fallen out of touch with Hattie herself. However, I thought about Hattie's situation and realised she had been extremely fragile for some months. There was her rejection of all types of food and drink by mouth, the night-time feeding tube with medication, and that deepening sleepiness. Sadly, I guessed poor Hattie must have died. Considering how strong our friendship had been, and what a lively mind she had, I knew she would have renewed our contact if things were otherwise.

Did Hattie have ME? My personal experience of the illness included a terrific amount of physical suffering but even though she was weak, sometimes disorientated and very forgetful, my friend was typically contented, so perhaps she didn't. She was disabled in many ways, but she wasn't in pain. She was very courageous and highly intelligent. My own illness and all the things that happened and affected me definitely taught me to be fully respectful and I will never dismiss someone's suffering, no matter what the cause might be.

* * *

I have thought about the power of a well-timed present; something that creates a feeling of joy. I wonder what it would have been like for me, if the door had opened to admit someone bearing an armful of cosy throws, bunches of flowers, or (more precious still) a nourishing meal all ready to reheat.

If my reader is a care giver who is doing those things for a sufferer, then your support is invaluable. The ill person is far more likely to recover if you help them, not less. Their relief and grateful thanks will be truly genuine, while they continue to long to be well and independent. Few people really want to be needy, and perhaps together you will plan ways of making that recovery come about.

Ideally, the ME victim would have support; it would be relentless, and it would be very kindly motivated. The fact is, with my writer's brain I certainly can imagine how I would have felt in that scenario, and all these years later it still makes me sad when I remember my vulnerability. I suspect my mother wanted to avoid a situation where I could rely on her help, but it was a harsh line to take. Others, including my husband, didn't seem to know what to do at all.

Still, many people do have steadfast helpers, and since some victims become so weak, they can't leave their bed then, in those instances, the support has to be put in place. Somehow, except for occasional periods of a few hours, I got out of my bed. There were times when I rolled to the edge, deliberately tipped myself off and landed on the floor, then crept very slowly out of my bedroom and down the narrow cottage staircase to do what I could with my day.

Kindness in itself is not always essential (and I'm the living proof) but how wonderful, if it is there. With energies depleted and resources almost wiped out, the ME patient deserves to be given any token, large or small, that shows someone is thinking about them. My Auntie Val sent the books and they were perfect. The happiness when I opened that unexpected parcel was indescribable. I felt real delight. Even better than that, I used the information they gave me in a positive way.

An appropriate gift which shows thought went into it, is a powerful kindness to anyone during a time of vulnerability, regardless of the cause. When my mother became gravely ill in 1996, I took small treats to tempt her appetite and I was not being disingenuous. Saddened by her illness and afraid for her, I hoped for the impossible, but cancer had taken hold. We couldn't beat it and when she passed away, I grieved deeply.

Nana

For many years after my recovery, I had a recurring dream. It was relentless, forcing my mind to revisit many familiar places in the Suffolk village where we lived when I was ill. In my dream, Nana was coming back to stay with us again and I walked over a broad village green, to stand on the corner and wait for her to arrive on a bus.

I think her departure must have been traumatic. I remember a sense of helplessness when she began to pack her bags, saying it was time for her to leave. In a psychological effect known as *fugue,* I lost the memory of those moments in any detail. (Dissociative fugue is said to be rare, but when events are very painful, in my experience it can affect someone in a way which does not indicate a deeper disorder.)

I'm not better! The phrase formed in my mind, although it remained unsaid. It was true. My condition was very poor. I was terribly miserable and all my movements were feeble. However, learning from many crushing put-downs I had received, I was reluctant to try to emphasise my situation and I knew I should be grateful for the help she had given me, so far.

So, I kept my thoughts to myself, even though I felt afraid of the future. I can recall her parting shot, which was cryptic and therefore rather unkind. "It's not easy, to have someone staying in your house ..."

I was sad. I loved her being in my house! I hadn't done anything wrong and, as a matter of fact, the route I was crawling along and beginning to understand was in line with some of her own beliefs.

"Potatoes are my passion!" Nana liked to declare, and it seemed a funny thing to say before the world opened up for me, with many realisations about good nutrition! Nana was a very well person, at eighty.

For many years, Nana's home was a tiny end terrace cottage in Shropshire. I saw her at regular intervals during the remainder of her life, which was long. We drove to visit her, or shared time at family gatherings and my children were always thrilled to see her.

She remained healthy and strong well into her eighties, keeping active with regular voluntary work in a hospital shop and enjoying visits from a friend who lived near her home. She loved cats but wouldn't keep one and explained that she needed to be free. A neighbour's black cat provided a spot of friendly company some-times, when he sat on Nana's kitchen windowsill and allowed him-self to be stroked. Occasionally, she went away on a holiday arranged by an organisation especially for elderly people.

It isn't always easy to manage the aging process in a positive way or retain a cheerful outlook, and I recognised the strength of char-acter my Nana possessed. I valued and admired her, but there had been that saddening element to our relationship. Most people who are obliged to live alone can describe the way in which activities break up the hours in a useful way, but a sense of loneliness has a way of returning and harming one's spirit. Nana could have stayed with us. My husband was kind towards her, and we loved her.

Why did she let herself get tired of me and the children, and leave before I was well? Was she irritated by my inactivity and my perceived failure to get moving? She went home to an empty house and her only pastimes during many hours alone were watching television and knitting. With every right to return to a quiet life, nevertheless her letters showed that her occasional excursions were few in reality, her friend visited just once a week and she often felt lonely and bored.

Of course, I'm conscious that my Nana was eighty years old, and the answer to my question may be very simple. Perhaps she was genuinely tired? In that case, it's possible she was too dignified to admit it!

Nana lived a long life. She continued energetic, youthful and smart until she was in her late eighties when fall down a flight of stairs in her cottage almost ended in disaster. Luckily my aunt found her in time to arrange for her to be treated in hospital and subsequently she was transferred to a care home. She went on, comfortable and alert during five or six more years when she needed to be nursed. Staff were kind, residents' rooms were full of light, with views of sweeping lawns, flowerbeds and trees, and Nana could sit by a picture window to watch birds fluttering around the feeders strung up for their benefit, and young squirrels playing there.

MY AUNT

My respect for my aunt was profound. When her later life brought the onset of an incurable degenerative illness and a sad passing, I missed her presence in my world. Sensible and practical, she had been important to me. She did something wonderful. She sent me a parcel. Any parcel, almost, as long as it was well-intentioned, would have felt wonderful and made me cry. Someone cared. Also, though, it was full of precious books and I was able to link my thoughts about joining the band of recovered ME sufferers with many ideas about good, effective nutrition.

My aunt was responsible for a change in my approach to good nutrition, and the start of thoughts and ideas which would bring about the difference in my life for which I longed. The day I received her bundle of books was springlike, but I had been feeling as if I was in a very dark tunnel. I was so lonely. At last, I saw something like a glimmer of light ahead. She included some of her own favourite books, as well as brand new ones chosen especially for me; her effort was inspired, and it made my heart fill with gratitude … and hope.

In itself, the gesture was supportive but, in addition, it immediately led to a link in my mind. That important message from the ME Association, something published in a pamphlet in those days, to the effect that there was recognition that those who achieve a recovery, or some partial recovery, tend to be people who paid attention to their diet.

Being believed was a giant relief. I was almost beaten flat, emotionally, as if I had been slapped, over and over again by harsh words, insults and turned backs. At last, something wonderful had happened.

After that, I was sure that Val really cared. She was a figure from my early childhood who used to share my parents' home in the first few years following their marriage and when I was a very small child. Still a teenager then, she used to take me out in my pram when I was a baby, or play with me in the garden of our home. We lived at the Langenhoe Lion, a public house near West Mersea, Essex. One of the group of people who surrounded me then, she seemed to have reappeared in similar guise. She always seemed nurturing and here she was, proving it surely? I trusted her.

There was a disappointment in store, when Val proved diffident about my thanks. After providing so much for me, with the kindness and the information I needed, at a later date she pointed out that my diaries might be chronicles of lived experience to me, but actually they were only my personal reflections! Even worse, ME (in her opinion) was not particularly monstrous when compared with some illnesses. So, there it was again, a certain disbelief! This time, from the person who helped me. She hadn't, after all, been able to comprehend how terribly ill and frightened I was, or how powerful the experience of illness and recovery had been for me.

Auntie Val's stroke of genius was never properly explained. I recovered and I subsequently tried to describe and discuss how I did it, and was quite surprised when she brushed off my comments and affected disinterest in my reflections. Both Val and my mother, Norma made efforts to alter their own diets a few years on from my recovery, looking for improved health (and taking a slightly baffling approach considering their stance before!) Norma got cross with the whole thing, missing cakes and other sweet treats. She abandoned the venture, not understanding that keeping the effort going for just a little longer might have led to her feeling refreshed. Val tired of it too, although she said her fingernails had been growing stronger so she supposed that was *something!*

Val always rejected any attempt on my part to thank her and it slowly became clear that she most definitely didn't accept that I had made myself better. I didn't challenge her. She had a friend whose daughter had suffered from ME for many years, and I wondered, would an acknowledgement of my recovery and my story somehow negate the long illness of her friend's daughter? Whatever the fundamental reason was, I valued the memory of what she did for me and I always will. When, so sadly, I lost one of my sons at the end of 2002, she came to stay, held my hand at first and seemed supportive. In later years, incredibly, she was unkind, saying things about my loss that showed she thought it meant my own life was thoroughly wrecked. It was a dangerous perception which shook my faith in life for a time, and almost wiped out my resolve to keep going and be courageous for the sake of my family. I needed to value and protect the lives of my other children. Again, I hung on to memories of her greatest efforts to help, and her fundamental honesty and good heartedness.

When it emerged that my aunt's friend (someone she had known from schooldays and who was her bridesmaid at her wedding in 1958) cared for an adult daughter who was weak and ill with ME, I wondered what my mother thought about that. My mother had been determined that I was malingering. Did she have an opinion about that unwell daughter (someone of my generation)? But conversation never touched on this during my mother's lifetime, nor on any other aspects of my illness. By the time the friend and her daughter came to my attention, Norma had gone and I was never to know the answer to my question.

Perhaps I learned lessons about people in general, to the effect that no-one is a saint! Often, we perceive according to what we need to understand and up to the limit we personally have for that understanding. Val needed to respect her best friend's beliefs, which she touched upon just once, in conversation with me. The daughter was so weak she could barely speak and the mother declared herself certain that one cannot make a change to the ME victim's condition. Sometimes, we create our own narrative.

ENVY, CRUELTY
AND DISSENT

When Nana left, I felt quite shaken. I wasn't sure what would happen next without the support she gave us or the daily structure which her presence and active help had created. How would I make our meals? Who would walk with my older son to the bus stop in the mornings? Little Andy wouldn't have an afternoon outing in his pushchair.

Those days were in advance of Auntie Val's generous parcel and the books were yet to be read, but I had begun to notice that eating well could give me a little more strength. Somehow, I muddled on. A neighbour became aware of Nana's disappearance and kindly helped with that early walk to the bus stop and back again later, and as the weather brought an occasional burst of early spring sunshine, I could sit outside in the fresh air and watch Andy play.

* * *

So many years have passed, I feel able to relate that I was a pretty young woman and the reason I refer to it is this. A beastly thing was happening, where envy caused other women to address my pallor and apparent weight gain with ill-concealed glee. (Actually, the extra weight was actually a false appearance caused by wearing two coats, I felt so cold!) Sometimes, very pretty women gather friends who openly admire them and an important, genuine friend to me was

Hattie who (at a later date) fell into this category. Too poorly to be competitive, she lived quietly and was content in her way. She complimented me and like me for myself.

Most attractive women know they will encounter copiers who are not straightforward. They appear in an outfit which exactly matches something you recently wore and if you mention you spotted it, you run into insults! You aren't supposed to identify the copying. My particular shade of auburn hair was often copied with colourant and I didn't mind (although it doesn't suit all skin tones!)

Then there are the envious people who try to put you down, looking for flaws. And of course, ill, pale, weak and just barely managing to dress myself, I was a target for that kind of untoward treatment. So, unfortunately, I came across people who actually insulted me and they did it to my face. They didn't care that they were turning on someone who was already down and I experienced being told I looked tired, older and ill.

Without apology, again, I refer to the lady who rejected my appeal for support. This memory always seems to hurt, and it stays very clear, too. As soon as I read her letter, I knew she was way off the point! I knew it in an objective way, and yet that didn't cushion the shock. I felt incredulous when her advice was to look at reasons "for the way you feel" and part of my incredulity was because I had explained myself. I did not feel unaccountably depressed as such. I was ill: too ill to live a normal life. I longed to get well. I was normally energetic and I wanted to be the same again! I was lumbered physically with something that was stopping me.

I sent her another letter in which I reiterated my points. I hung on to my good manners but then, when another response came, it was as if she got annoyed with me and carried away by her own ideas. Full of affected knowledge and cruelly defiant, its content could only be described as cheeky.

"I read all the articles and look at research and I'm not convinced this is a physical illness!"

"Ugh!" I thought. It was a lofty stance. I saw no excuse for it and I would not permit further damage to my pride. I left her alone after that.

The agony aunt wasn't the only person who thought my vulnerability gave her licence to declare that I should look into my *behaviour* to find out why I felt so weak. Some people will highlight achievements of others as if the ME victim needs aspirations, when the truth is, they long to get up and begin to do all the things they miss so much. Dissent is cruel but the ME sufferer must remember those who take that stance, affecting some knowledge, are in reality highly unlikely to have any. They do not want to be asked for help but they pretend they have every reason; you must do it alone for your own good.

I knew my mother was saying I was *just depressed* (as if that were not in itself a cause for alarm), taking a stance about it, thinking I had to somehow pull myself together and deliberately ignoring all my signs of physical illness.

There are those who may never have been faced with the sort of nightmare you've plunged into, and they might deliberately ignore your desperation and your need to seek any route to recovery. They might make a remark which is a type of accusation, and it isn't fair. They say, if a nutritional approach takes care of it, then no way is it a real illness. In that event, I would point out that in cases of heart disease, obesity, fatty liver, diabetes, some lung disorders, migraine and more, we know the patients are often significantly helped by lifestyle and health changes.

There is no reason to allow anyone to suggest you were not ill after the nutritional approach brings an improvement.

What if your dissenter proposes that, if some people recover in a way the medical world would label spontaneous, the whole thing, especially when it is prolonged, has to be imaginary, even when others (like me) struggled through a recovery process? On this, I believe you have a right to say (if you want to answer and argue at all) *So, what?* Perhaps that was true of those people. It's been harder for you, and you are entitled to approach your health your way. You may offer no answer for the conundrum because, quite simply it's not your responsibility.

In my first book No Medals for ME, I explained that a helper who was paid to come and do my housework, was a great comfort. She was a good person who gave the household her best efforts, and she never said anything unkind to me. I was beginning to find my way forward by then and I was determined to keep on trying, but I had been very hurt and the support Evelyn brought was a blessing. I genuinely felt a surge of strength from the emotional gain. The ME victim who seems stronger after being comforted should never be mistrusted. With the comfort and kindness that is so desperately needed, there can result a small sense of wellbeing. If someone is prepared to help, working together they and the patient might build on that emotional development and welcome improvement.

OTHER TYPES OF ILLNESS

Influenza (the flu)

Over the years I have fallen ill with strains of influenza twice. The first time, a single mother by then, I sent a muddled text message to my eldest son, who (to his credit) deciphered it and came at once. My other children were in their early teens. I was so feverish, I lost track of time and I remember how strange it was, when I woke up feeling much better on the third day to find my son, then in his twenties, reclining calmly beside me wearing his skinny jeans and boots, with his long red hair falling over his shoulders, waiting and watching until I recovered. I felt as if I had returned from another world and yet, in a conundrum typical of ME, on that occasion its symptoms didn't crowd in! One might wonder, why not? To me, it doesn't matter.

Another flu-related episode was much nastier, bringing overtones of resentment from a group of people who were definitely subject to pack mentality. Inevitably, the experience was reminiscent of ME.

At the start of 2018, I fell ill and became feverish with aches in all my joints and a cough. This illness seemed to be some kind of virus and the worst of the symptoms went on for about seven days. After I began to improve, I stopped feeling hot and miserable from coughing but I was in a condition of post viral exhaustion. It wasn't a return of ME and wasn't anything like that level of suffering, but it was a debilitating effect that floored me for several more weeks.

I was registered on a course in a local college and felt disappointed when I couldn't possibly return at the start of the spring term. It seemed fortunate that I had begun the course mainly for my own enjoyment, and in fact already knew the topics very well. I had sufficient education in counselling but, when I registered, I thought it would be enjoyable to share some days in a learning environment. I looked forward to adding a new certificate to my portfolio. I was a mature learner, older than a handful of my classmates but not very much older than some.

An essay was required under the heading of *Equality and Diversity*. At home, with my mind feeling much better in advance of my bodily recovery, I looked up some work I had presented in a similar course. I carefully amended and typed up an assignment, and submitted it online. I made sure my document matched the brief, and although it was an early submission, I reasoned that this was unlikely to matter. Being late is something that generally causes the most trouble with tutors! I enjoyed this positive action, made the document smart with page numbers and headings and a neat layout, and I thought to look engaged with the process, showing my determination to remain a hardworking member of the study group.

About five weeks after the term began, I was at a point where I could contemplate travelling back to the college. I felt fragile, but I packed a lunch, snacks and bottles of water, deciding I would aim to stay for one morning and see how things went. I was rather proud of myself when I entered the warm hallway of the university centre building. I had coped with the bus ride, which took an hour, and felt ready for the day ahead. I heard the hum of voices from students who gathered as usual near the foot of the staircase, and there was the good scent of coffee which always emanated from the tiny café near the reception area. I joined the group.

I felt surprised when only one or two of my classmates were friendly.

"She's back!" One cheerful person announced but others made no comment. No-one asked how I felt. The tutors were oddly cool, too. There seemed to be a general sense that it was too late, I had missed too much work and lost my footing amongst them all.

The social experiences I'd gone through years before had shaped me in a way, and I wasn't expecting or wishing for praise on my return. In retrospect, the comparison with my efforts to slide back into life after ME was there; however, it was not at the top of my mind. Instead, I was hopeful as ever. I would have been encouraged by a welcome of some kind! Inevitably, I felt disappointed when I sensed their resentment, which was a shade more obvious than disinterest and rather unpleasant.

What's this all about? I wondered. Was it supposed to be the case that I had stayed away deliberately, and now I shouldn't return? I reviewed my communications over the past month or so, and knew, in fact, I had kept the administration team (and therefore the course tutors) updated.

Then I learned that my careful essay was not going to be awarded any marks at all!

"Zero?" I echoed, when a tutor informed me of this.

"Because you missed classes! This isn't an online course, you know!" She was hostile.

I was astonished. The study history I had described to university centre interviewers was chronicled in a portfolio, and it clearly proved my prior learning in topics to be included during this course. I made no secret of the fact that I had a number of certificates already; I was proud of my achievements, and I could have been respected for them. I certainly wasn't expecting there would be a problem.

I saw it as a straightforward situation. I had paid for my place on the course; I knew the syllabus already; I was fully respectful of the tutors (who were mostly my juniors) and I was absolutely prepared to do my best and enjoy myself at the same time.

However, following the rebuff I spent time in deep thought. I went over and over some of my experiences in the college, and I recalled a few sharp comments which had simply seemed odd at the time. There came a better understanding of the treatment I received, and a few things fell into place.

It was a fact that I knew the subject matter of the assignment in question very well, having conducted my own workshops on a related topic! Observational psychology, with linked issues of equality and diversity, was (and remains) particularly interesting to me. I had certainly spotted some resentment from tutors during the first term, especially those who were younger than me, and I knew that we were all in an awkward position, in a way, since students on a counselling course are continually asked to offer feedback and when I was asked for my comments, I couldn't help seeming well-informed. Nevertheless, students' responses to the subjects are supposed to be welcomed, so the tutors did not cover themselves with glory by being so obviously irritated by my presence!

To put me firmly in my place, my liking for online study was deemed a fault. There had been gossip and there followed an accusation. I must have tired of being present in classes, decided the team, and I had surely faked illness so that I could study in my preferred way, at home. Online studies were wrongly linked with my absence and this perception led to me being viewed with suspicion.

My work would not be marked! I was given to understand that I had underestimated my capabilities and (it seemed) I couldn't possibly know the subject. Later in the year, I was required to provide that assignment as part of my collection of submissions overall, and once again I deliberated carefully. Was there any truth in the idea that I had misunderstood the assignment? I thought not, and decided to present the very same document. Feeling defiant, I changed the date and that was all! Was anyone astute enough to spot the identical essay? I'll never know, but it gained a pass mark because there was nothing wrong with it as a reflection of my understanding of the course module.

Narrow-minded suspicion had its foundations in aspects of envy (because I knew the subject so well) but also it was familiar from the days when ME affected me. It seemed to be connected with that problem that some people have when they are unable to comprehend that you are taking a long time to get well. My illness had been used as something to hold against me in a setting where I was already poorly received by people who felt challenged by my prior learning. Since I had begun to make friends with some class-mates before the episode, I suspected the tutors had also affected the perceptions of those students who became cool towards me. At a later date, a few discreet enquiries led to the discovery that this was true. There had been discussions about me, with encour-agement from those tutors who had their own agenda. With the excuse that trainees in counselling were entitled to reflect on the character and behaviour of one other, an adverse picture of my actions was established.

I forced myself to be philosophical about this treatment as far as anyone could see. My hurt feelings were hidden. In reality, I *was* quite offended! I didn't return to the course with an air of bravado and I didn't need a pat on the back, but I found the resentment painful, as anyone would. I cannot respect those who turn away from someone on the basis of their own perceptions (or another's) instead of looking for a proper understanding, especially when their whole ethos is supposed to be the very opposite!

After all, the ill person is the one who is most entitled to hate their condition and resent that long time spent virtually idle, as well as the subsequent debilitation with all its problematic issues. In order to rebuff accusations of weakness however, one ends up hav-ing to be extra brave and it can be a challenge to hold on to those hopes for a good outcome in every situation.

* * *

A Medical Misdiagnosis

Life managed to throw a serious medical upset at me when I was in my early fifties. I felt slightly unwell when I got a skin rash but the greatest cause for alarm was its appearance, since lesions were very sore and multiplied at a frightening rate. They were painful, and looked unsightly. I sought medical help, was not treated sympathetically, and it wasn't long before I realised the shared responses of a local doctor and a dermatologist seemed incredibly odd. There was that worrying, suspicious attitude again, and an unaccountable wish to force me to take tranquillisers! I refused.

This time, it seemed absolutely logical for me to receive clinical care, including vital blood tests. Rashes were appearing and multiplying on my body almost as I watched, and it was nightmarish. Still, I was rejected. In fact, I was even made to feel small when I insisted on seeing my local doctors again following their initial rejection. They gave me a prescription for a topical cream and except for raising the issue of tranquillisers again, that was all.

My attempts to secure more comprehensive treatment were deflected for many weeks, during which time I tried to buy into their instructions to relax and wait for the rashes to disappear. I was terribly confused. Couldn't they see what was happening to my skin? I felt sick too, and became somewhat thin.

There was no spontaneous change; in fact, the condition of my skin worsened and after some months I was quite an ill person all over again. While I sickened and weakened, increasingly I felt sure there was something strange about all this.

A number of insulting comments were made by a female GP, who would not offer me treatment when I called in distress one day. She said, I may as well go to the emergency department of the local hospital. By this time, I knew for certain there was something unusual going on and it wasn't in my favour. When she told me that I would never recover unless I stopped making myself ill, I caught sight of my reflection in the hall mirror, saw my own shocked face, and it was a defining moment. I was being profoundly failed.

I made a formal application for sight of my medical records, with a patient's entitlement under the Data Protection Act. There was considerable argument against this (argument which, I'm now aware, is not permissible) and at the hospital the consultant's secretary wanted to sit opposite me while I read the material in her presence. She had no right to do so, but it didn't matter. Ignoring her, I read the documents and realised it wasn't surprising that my interest caused alarm. I found the team had chosen to state I had a mental disorder: not because I had ME in my history but because I was a bereaved mother.

In reality, I was brave about my sad loss. It was very painful to find I was labelled psychotic because of a tragedy which, presumably, the medical professionals couldn't contemplate anyone bearing without mental harm. I had been living a positive, fulfilling life since my loss. I was often deeply sad and reflective but I took care of myself and my surviving children. I was not psychotic.

At least I knew what had happened to hold up my recovery! Quickly, I sought a second opinion from a different dermatologist and gained access to a hospital in another part of the country. In his surgery, everything I had suffered began to change.

When a nurse saw that I was shaking with anxiety she got me a glass of water, but no-one suggested my poor condition was the result of anxiety. Of course, I felt scared because I dreaded being denied care again. However, whereas the first dermatologist only saw me privately and refused to examine me, this time I was treated respectfully and correctly. This doctor was honourable and my consultation was conducted in the presence of the nurse, who remained calmly at my side and held my hand during a thorough examination.

This consultant concentrated on my actual condition as I presented in his surgery and it was only a few minutes before he identified a form of anaemia which, thankfully, would respond to a range of essential medications. He ordered clinical tests to back up this information. Treated impartially and correctly, I got well.

This experience revived some of the old hurt and confusion, as well as creating more. I had been fed conflicting information for many months, and when my eyes were opened after reading the medical files, I saw approaches had been ingratiating and falsely soothing. I had been recommended to use weak, topical creams and try not to worry. I had been treated like a fool. The suppurating rash (which even smothered my back, where I couldn't reach even if I had wanted to scratch my skin) was supposed to be self-inflicted and a small group of medical people had arranged for a presumptive diagnosis of *psychosis* to be entered in my records. With my liking for research, before long I looked up the mental affliction I was supposed to have, and felt both horrified and astonished. Obviously, the times when I had expressed feelings of distress had been used against me. Notes had been made to try to undermine my appearance of mental and emotional stability and I had been forced into a category (self-harming) which made no sense under the circumstances.

This was a fight with the medical profession, and I did need their help. They had a role and I battled to get the care I needed to make a recovery. It was tough. Within copies of my personal medical records, I found lies, masses of them. A framework had been created initially by the shared endeavour of a GP and a dermatologist, then forced forward in the attempt to prove the initial, ill-conceived mistake.

There was even a frightening remark. *We will wait and see what happens with interest!* At a later date I questioned this, and the doctor who wrote it into the record denied its sinister implications and insisted it simply revealed a kindly interest. This could not have been the case, since clinical investigations had been withheld at that time.

I would like to refer back to my earlier comments about pointless argument. When the argument is obviously facile, I'd maintain that it's best ignored. It probably doesn't matter; you can refuse to be harmed, make no comment and rise above it. When other people imagine they are better than you, it's often only their perception and their frame of reference may be limited. If you notice someone is spouting lofty rubbish, there may be no need to take it on board!

This new experience was a different matter.

A pharmacist who knew me was shown the dermatologist's initial prescription. I had already made up my mind that the proposed medication was inappropriate. The pharmacist remained professional and he didn't interfere as such, but he asked a question that spoke volumes. Was I going to throw the prescription away? It was a question founded on wisdom rather than levity. The harm that was about to be perpetuated on my medical history (if I accepted medication for non-existent psychosis) was obvious to anyone who took an intelligent approach to my situation.

Certainly, I would bin the prescription. I hadn't spent a minute thinking I should take pills I didn't need! There was no question of it, and there was definitely a case for completely ignoring such non-sense … and yet, I knew it would remain unchallenged on my medical records if I did nothing. Also, I risked going forward with continued illness left untreated.

The dermatologist had made an error and I suspect he knew that within a very short time, but it was followed by ruthless self-inter-est. His behaviour intensified and further comments about my mental health were added to my records before I gained access and read them. Then, I saw, he was afraid to lose face. His assumption of superiority was a result of his blinkered self-belief, and he was copied because other medical professionals who surrounded him also believed in this. As an individual, he didn't matter actually; I maintain that belief on a personal level because he wasn't right. But he was unprofessional and he failed me and harmed my medical records, which would have been a dreadful outcome if I hadn't sought a second opinion and recovered. His actions couldn't be ignored. I did have to address the false medical history he created, for all the reasons I've described.

From my consultation with a new dermatologist to a point when an obvious feeling and appearance of real recovery took place, the process took just about two weeks. In the hands of the first dermatologist who, with extraordinary hubris, chose to abandon clinical care and dabble in a spot of psychology he didn't really understand, I had been ill and denied chances to recover for ten months. It was an intense and dangerous episode, not only the fault of the dermatologist but also of those who sought to back him up. They were subject to effects of pack mentality and also had their own interests to protect. I am glad to say, I turned anger into action. I made a formal complaint, insisted upon a letter of apology, and was awarded a sum in compensation for the shocking failure in clinical care.

It was, after all, an experience that highlighted how a medical team can sometimes be expected to help, and when that help is appropriate it's an absolute right. For instance, some ME victims might ask a doctor to consider the possibility that they might be anaemic or have a different fundamental condition. It does show that a patient must not give up seeking wellness. Perhaps you have to input as much as *you* can, then also seek more and be relentless when it becomes essential to ask for your right to a full examination and a clear outcome.

In a strange conundrum, sometimes it seems that medically trained professionals who have studied for so long still end up with a certain lack of understanding. They form ideas, and sometimes those are depressingly without positivity, or oddly misplaced, even morbid. They can seem contemptuous of their patients. A request to check one's medical records can bring an enlightening insight if this happens.

Naturally, I must qualify these observations (which stem from real experience) with the fact that many medically trained professionals only mean well, and generally do their best to help their patients.

COURAGE

In 2002 I was forty-eight years of age. I was very busy every day, a mother of five by this time with my first son being twenty-one and the youngest just six. In a completely unexpected turn of events, I lost one of my sons. Andy, my baby in the first book, met with an accident. The full, heart-breaking history is not for this book but I will say that I believe I then proved two important things about ME and they are closely linked.

First, although I was in an agony of sorrow, I didn't collapse with symptoms. Feeling shocked and full of grief was inevitable and that depth of pain can lead to a form of exhaustion or even a feeling of sickness, but it didn't make the condition of ME resurface. ME isn't a direct result of emotional pain or sorrow.

Second, I had courage. I kept going because I knew I had to support, encourage and motivate Andy's brothers and his sister. Courage isn't in question, in an ME sufferer.

It's a difficult fact, and I already learned the hard way that human beings often find it impossible to recognise courage in another unless it's somehow obvious (a mountain rescue perhaps?) Some years on from my dreadful loss, I met those resentful tutors in a college course where they disliked my wisdom, experience and prior learning, none of which I could conceal, nor did I want to.

When I became uncomfortable with a role play session one day,

I pointed out that person-centred counsellors need to be respectful, not plough on with a topic of conversation when a client who is very sad indicates they cannot bear it. For this input and my considered explanation, I received inappropriate censure from people who had never faced or crossed the hurdles I had. They tried to raise a question over my personal strength and resolve but they were misguided and their efforts only underlined the paucity of the course and tuition, and the way trainees failed to understand many of the important theories they needed to learn.

For unkind things to say, there's a remark commonly made to bereaved mothers which can't be beaten.

I don't know how you cope. I couldn't.

This is an insult disguised as a compliment. Incredibly unkind, with cruel implications, it's the most unwelcome comment I've ever been unlucky enough to receive. Extraordinarily often, I have found myself in a position where someone thinks they may deliver themselves of this remark and (of course) they mean: *how can you carry on, considering your loss?*

Perhaps a natural expression of incredulity is understandable to some extent, and it's born of blissful ignorance of how it really feels to lose a child and the challenges that follow. I don't think those facts excuse it. Yes, it's almost impossible to find a way forward, but I had a right to try. The second part of the sentence (*I couldn't*) is an attempt to create a distance, but what does this imply? That since the bereaved parent finds their path and they can carry on, then they are different from other parents and possess a harder, less feeling nature?

So, would this speaker really give up in the face of unbearable grief? What if, like me, they had a family of brothers and sisters of the lost child, who all depended on their mother and father to keep going, to be brave, and to find ways to show them that their own lives still matter? To give them comfort, and look for the good in life? What kind of message would I have offered my precious surviving children, if I had seemed to find no further point in anything?

In any context, before saying something spiteful, people need to remember:

There, but for the grace of God, I go.

Pale Faces

Above, under the heading My Beliefs, I discussed the pale faces featured in some articles about ME. It's a sad fact that pictures of ill people make others turn away. Also, unfortunately, they can make sufferers feel hopeless.

Pictures of people looking weak don't help the cause and they don't work to convince others of the extent of an ME patient's suffering. Perhaps this doesn't seem to make sense, but generally they don't engender pity in an observer who knows nothing about the effects of ME.

Such images also reinforce sufferers' shared belief that there is no escape from being a typical ME victim. So, it's toxic, in my opinion, for the ME sufferer to concentrate on looking so ill.

I think it's essential to teach yourself to cherish your individuality and the freedom to look forward to better times. You haven't *got to be* the same. Sufferers write about how horrible it is to suffer with ME symptoms. Many are photographed looking wan, with that ME pallor and a tired face, for any article about the illness.

Of course, it's a fact that the pictures tell a story and it can be fascinating to read about the experience another has had when it feels similar to one's own, but there are pitfalls in this overall picture, even when it presents the truth. It's important not to identify with other people to the greatest possible extent. Instead, see

132

yourself as an individual. This is a unique illness in that it can have varying symptoms and there isn't a medical cure, but you can try to make yourself hopeful.

Someone has suffered from ME for thirty years? Why? Settling into illness, believing there is no option, can have a false comfort: yes, other sufferers know what you are going through, and yes, it seems, from their stories, that you have no need to demand anything of yourself … but that way, you have little hope of making a recovery!

The fascinating, useful and scientific details about how vitamins can work for the human body have been available for a very long time. If it's known that deficiency causes certain ailments, look for those in yourself as an ME sufferer, don't succumb to despair, and start to boost your vitamin intake. Really believe in yourself as someone who can get well.

* * *

While I was preparing this book for publication, something happened which underlined my feeling that ME sufferers may unwittingly fail to help themselves. It's a sad example of the perception that defines an ME sufferer as part of a whole section of society, a vast group with which they identify more than any other, and the danger that lies in that perception.

I read an article in a magazine from a contributor who suffers from ME. They proposed that people who felt unhappy about being confined and separated from society and their usual routines during the pandemic were not thoughtful. This is putting it mildly, since the writer used powerful vocabulary and the piece was an abusive diatribe focused against the entire rest of the population as opposed to those with ME. Those who were struggling in lockdown were labelled selfish and worse. Those who put on their masks and went out for their shopping were (unbelievably) termed *disease spreading, able-bodied people.*

It wasn't hard to understand the writer's intended message. It's tough to be made to stay at home, blocked from the things you love to do, and while many people were only forced to be that way because of the coronavirus, ME sufferers are often even less able to control their lives. As an ME sufferer myself I got the message, but its delivery was out of control. Some who suffered especially as a result of being locked down had mental and emotional problems. People with obsessional afflictions were more constrained and many types of illness, disability, or other suffering such as loneliness were made worse. Families where there was abuse were forced into situations where they were more unhappy, even in danger.

While I firmly believe the ME sufferer is entitled to feel and express the emotions that come with it (and many of those are certainly linked with the attitudes they come across) it's never going to be helpful to look resentful and full of pointless anger, or adopt an attitude that makes others think, *goodness! Why do you feel so much more entitled to attention than everyone else?* Plenty of people in the rest of the world have their problems and also have to find courage.

CONCLUSION

I returned to live in Essex again in 1991, after my freedom from debilitating illness was almost certain.

Neither of my parents would ever talk about that long illness and I know my recovery was supposed to be spontaneous. They are gone and they are sorely missed. My mother was fun and funny when she was with her grandchildren and her creative ability was enormous. The sketches, paintings and needlework she left behind are treasured. Her legacy of artistic brilliance lies firmly within my adult children who are designers, artists and tattooists.

My father was much respected in his operatic group. He became an active elderly gentleman, who enjoyed walking, gardening and cooking. A wine connoisseur, he would take me out to dinner regularly and appeared to take more interest in me as time went on. Cognitive dissonance? I was able to enjoy his company *in the moment,* at last.

I have been well most of the time. Essentially, I returned to my naturally energetic and cheerful self. I rode again and enjoyed both hacking in the countryside and taking horses through their paces in indoor schools. I had more children. I walked, trained dogs for myself and other people, and studied. I returned to experiencing how joyful life can be.

On taking good health for granted, perhaps this seems incredible but when I look back over the years since my recovery, I know I have been capable of assuming I'll stay well. I just wanted to get on with things. When the pandemic hit the world in 2020, one son pointed out that I needed to be very careful. "Mum, you'd crumple up like a paper bag …!" I was careful and I eventually accepted the vaccine after much deliberation.

In a respectful note about long covid, so-called, I would mention this. If I had to start all over again, to regain my health and recover from the (surely similar) condition now known as long covid; I would be looking at the same approaches. I would use my method for recovering from ME.

Sometimes I have overestimated my strength and endurance, and joining kickboxing aerobics was really silly. I didn't realise how strenuous the class was, until I was in the middle of it! I stopped jumping around and air kicking, made my apologies and left. I was a little embarrassed, but as a matter of fact that type of exercise didn't suit me at all! It was very undignified! At least I didn't get terribly ill.

I was honest about my reluctance to risk my energies, but the leader of the class didn't miss an opportunity to make a sly remark. "Oh … an ME sufferer!" She said it with a certain rude emphasis and a raised eyebrow, but I let her attitude slide off my consciousness although, clearly, I noticed it.

There were times when ailments such as a viral sore throat or a tummy bug affected me harshly during the first few years after I made my significant recovery, and even nowadays the occasional shaky episode will occur when I am very tired. This makes it important to return to my way of healthy living, if I have lapsed.

I retained my fascination with good health and I had well and truly learned the lessons I found in my research. I knew my recovery was a scientific process. I also found a determination to care for myself as much as possible, as opposed to turning to medical teams, and this served me well during that illness in later life, when my condition was prolonged by medical misdiagnosis at a time when I really did need clinical care.

Some people change so much, they become fitness fanatics in every way. They discover a new world in terms of food and fitness, turn everything around and enjoy it. They may decide not to eat sugar, drink alcohol or caffeinated tea and coffee *ever again*.

However, some of my happier childhood times affected me as time went on. Never to be forgotten was the comforting nature of our meals, which were home-cooked and tasty. I enjoy baking and I like sweet treats, so, as long as I am feeling well in general, I include some sugar in my diet. In terms of physical activity, with my recovery came the ability to be quite active but since that is my natural tendency, I have overestimated my energy on many occasions. I don't fall back into ME when this happens, but I get warning migraine headaches. I have enjoyed using a gym, riding horses and running around after my children, but I'm never going to be a mountaineer, or even a jogger!

* * *

There is no fairy-tale magic wand, or incredible invention of new medicine, to be swallowed in a pill or received via a vaccine against ME. It takes courage to let go of that longing for it to be a disease with a cure. But, drawing on the ideas about psychology (sufferers, nay-sayers and so on) and the nutritional method I've described, is there any way you can do what I did, and care less about what it actually is and more about your way out of the mire, on a route to recovery?

And yet, with a different perception, is there actually some kind of magic for ME? Yes, I'm sure there is, and it's in nutrition and in your effort. It's your spell and you can make it.

So, when some people argue against the credibility of my story I have to say, *so what?* It happened as I told it. There's no need to be offended by the idea that the unconscious mind could have been affected by the general perceptions amongst ME sufferers and those who take an interest *(a disease process, no way out except when medical people invent a pill ...)* Instead, abandoning any sense of having a point to prove, an open mind can lead to the potential to recover. What you can do, brings a certain magic after all.

Postscript

Challenges, reflections, looking back, looking ahead

I listened to a radio interview with a swimmer, and she was explaining her reasons for battling the seas to swim very long distances. She acknowledged the risks, including drowning in stormy weather, or perishing of cold. There was another risk, too. For goodness' sake, she could have been stung, she said, by a type of jellyfish that's so poisonous, it kills a human being instantly!

Why does anyone knowingly go into such a situation? I know people do, and many activities which humans throw themselves into are dangerous. Yet, life will find your challenges for you. If you are lucky enough to be healthy, this is surely something to cherish!

The ME sufferer longs, first and foremost, to regain strength and wellbeing. The intensity and the misery are unlikely to promote any intention of finding a snowy mountain to climb or a wild sea to swim across! However, that person is not naturally fainthearted. In reality, they may be one of the most courageous people one could ever meet.

My long-ago confusion disappeared with better understanding. I examined my experiences in the light of psychology and psychodynamic theories, and I thoroughly reviewed them all and learned that I was not to blame for the treatment I suffered. My fear of being disbelieved has gone, because it doesn't matter. I got well, and

I became mentally strong. However, I avoid casual conversations about ME because like most people, I really don't like being unfairly presented with pointless argument, especially when it's about something that matters so much, to me. Conversation in-depth, I welcome, as long as I am given the chance to explain my thoughts.

Reflections are subjective and they don't mean I didn't care. The opposite was true, or why would I have felt so hurt? I was subjected to spite from people whom I loved. It wasn't possible to go on as if nothing had happened, although one of the strangest feelings was that awareness that some people thought I could. I know I became determined to safeguard myself better, after I regained my health.

Since life does present challenges to us all in time, none of the folk who were cruel to you (the ME sufferer) will have a charmed life free from any form of suffering. For sure, they will have to confront unhappiness. What goes around comes around and, sadly, seeing others go through tough times themselves is inevitable. With compassion, I don't feel relief from my own burden when troubles arise for others. In any case, I'm always unable to voice a comparison with my experience, partly because it was (and still is) negated by the disbelief and partly because … well … how could I? I can't force others to understand (and if they didn't believe me when I was obviously ill, those same people won't give me credibility now!)

There's no comfort in knowing that the disbelievers will encounter their own issues at some point in their lives, but it's a fact that the ME survivor's ability to empathise is likely to have its limits! That's understandable. Perhaps they won't actually make the connection between their past behaviour and your reservations. You might, though.

Looking ahead? Of course, you must, and be hopeful and positive. Get the nutrition right, increase what you can do as and when the real ability to move forward happens. Trust yourself above anyone else, especially if they are trying to force you to be active when you know it's a crazy idea.

AUTHOR'S NOTES
AND REFERENCES

With reference to the two main books which I turned to, I'm aware that I used them a long time ago and I would like to preclude the list with an explanation. Why do I stick to these, to discuss what I did and offer suggestions?

Some modern changes are good. Others may be open to question. For instance, I had five children. Would I ever have placed a new baby to sleep in crib or pram, lying on their back? Never! Nor would I want to, now. However, it's the advice given by health visitors to modern mothers. But all my babies did well, and so do the vast majority of new babies! My point is: there can be merit found in old ways, and modern too. You just have to use ideas judiciously and thoughtfully.

Dr Mackarness' book, Not All in the Mind absolutely grabbed my attention. I read it all through and I knew that, even then, there were some who criticised its theories. Now, I tend to notice that masked food allergy gets referenced as a contentious theory, much as ME is habitually referenced as a mystery in that irritating, copying approach I've described.

It was so important to let go of a certain mindset, a belief that my situation was hopeless, and a slavish set of thoughts which most ME sufferers can certainly be forgiven for picking up from the material they are offered.

However, the doctor was obviously able to help patients and for me the book provided valuable information. I used it, but didn't necessarily follow every point without very careful consideration of my personal responses. I definitely found that three- or four-days' abstinence from a food I was eating repetitively led to withdrawal symptoms on the second and third days, followed by a feeling of freshness which was very welcome (and in that sense I stuck closely to the plan) but I also found that I could then return to the same food in small quantities, sometimes.

I also came to understand myself and how my own system responds to various foods, with very careful attention to my diet diary.

Regarding The Vitamins Explained Simply, it has pieces of information inside which are pure gold for an ME sufferer and they should leap off the page and be understood. For example: the intake often needs to be more, when you are ill. Details of how certain deficiencies affect the body. I found it electrifying to see how certain ailments which I was actually suffering might be treated with attention to my vitamin intake, and when I sought to rectify the situation, it worked!

References:
Books (non-fiction)

The Vitamins Explained Simply Revised and Extended by Leonard Mervyn BSc PhD FRSC Prepared and produced by the Editorial Committee (Science of Life Series)

Not All in the Mind by Dr Richard Mackarness published by Pan Books Ltd.

No Medals for ME by Lisette Skeet published by the Strategic Book Publishing and Rights Co. USA | Singapore www.sbpra.net

* * *

Quotes:

"A thousand knees, ten thousand years together

Naked Fasting upon a barren mountain

and still Winter, in storm perpetual

Could not move the gods to look that way thou wert" W. Shakespeare (The Winter's Tale)

"Let food be thy medicine and medicine be thy food!"

Hippocrates

Further Reflections

For readers who enjoy aspects of psychology and behaviour.

Cognitive Dissonance and Congruence

Cognitive dissonance: you are uncomfortably aware of a problem with your words or actions and the way in which it affects you, since it may not align with your fundamental beliefs.

Congruence: you are true to yourself and strive to be honest with others.

Of course, the two concepts are linked. In a state of cognitive dissonance, you probably know where congruence lies but circumstances affect your ability to achieve it. In true congruence, honesty is achieved, although it could still be painful since it may lead to change.

A Barbeque

Towards the end of the summer of 1989, I was invited to a family gathering. I was happy to accept and excited by the prospect of an outing. It was a sunny day and my two small boys would be able to play with their cousins in a beautiful country garden.

I had made significant changes to my state of health but I was fairly fragile, and I carried a shooting stick for something to lean on and to use, occasionally, as a seat. I climbed out of the car and my

144

husband and children were by my side when we met a gathering of around fifteen people, standing on a gravelled area behind the old Post Office. Jonathan and Andrew ran ahead of me; my husband entered into a conversation with another guest at once and I made my way into the garden.

No-one remarked on my arrival or the fact that it was many months since I had been able to visit my family and I was conscious of a most extraordinary feeling from the start. I wasn't brought a drink or something to eat from the long tables which had been set up on the lawns, and although the barbeque was wonderful and the drinks table was loaded with bottles and gleaming glassware, whilst other guests could easily collect what they needed, I was shaky, and would have benefitted from help. It seemed to go unnoticed that the shooting stick was essential but also created some difficulty in helping myself to food.

Even worse, no-one said it was lovely to see me! My long, awful experience was ignored. It's true that people often simply don't know what to say or how to behave in relation to something they know nothing about, but … that weird silence … it made me wonder, was I not worth more than this? Was anyone glad I was there, after all? I wasn't even sure of that!

I had a strange childhood with many important issues neglected. As an adult who longed to talk about how I felt, at first, I was confused again. However, I think I must have seen how it would be that day and recognised the silence, and remembered past failures to acknowledge me for the person I was. It led to making a decision, and it was deliberate: I would carry on and let that be the way things were. My children deserved to play with their cousins. It was a kind of game of *make pretend*. I had to pretend I wasn't much altered.

This was the start of my experience of **cognitive dissonance,** wanting to revisit my family but hurting because they recognised me only as the person I once was, caring nothing for the life-changing events that affected me. It's no wonder I sometimes got cross in later years, over family issues which were unrelated to my illness and yet revived memories of being side-lined. I was to study psychological processes in the more distant future but at the time, I was just living through the things that affected me. I didn't want to make painful changes.

The Value of Counselling

I have presented a detailed examination of the way in which some people treat an ME victim, and I have discussed the awful struggle I was left with, when I couldn't find compassion in those around me; not even those who might have been expected to care. I had many thoughts and feelings I would have liked to express but they were hidden over years. It would have been beneficial to me, to go forward honestly.

I know some ME victims receive a good deal of attention to their mental health. It's valuable to talk about feelings, whatever the cause of an upset is, but when I think about the harm an uninformed counsellor might be capable of inflicting upon an ME victim, I am sure that counselling sessions in a formal setting need to be postponed while the patient is ill and debilitated. I maintain this, even though I experienced a need to talk. When strength permits, a person-centred counsellor who can demonstrate a good understanding of the therapeutic process is the one to find. A psychodynamic counsellor who trained in higher education could be helpful post recovery, with sessions concentrating on events retrospectively, and I'd recommend looking for someone whose training encompassed, at the very least, the three-year term of a degree and ideally far longer in an excellent university setting.

It was partly the fault of the tutor that all the students who were present when I described something of ME maintained their impression that it is essentially a mental health issue. Some, I suspected of failing to pay any attention at all. It seemed to me they would let the discussion slip away from their thoughts as soon as possible. They had *not* listened carefully, even though, if they planned to be counsellors, paying close attention was supposed to be their main priority!

The episode underlined several things. How an important aspect of counselling and therapy must be the presence of emotional intelligence (EI) which unfortunately cannot be readily acquired. There needs to be a foundation of EI as a character trait, to develop and enhance during the learning process. How simply having an affectation of *saviour mentality* isn't good enough. The paucity of understanding that existed as a general problem, endemic in that study environment (even though that would appear to be a contradiction in terms!) People who wish to go forward to support and counsel others need to be equipped with the best possible personal awareness and a real sense of excellence.

Above everything else they aim to do for their clients, therapists and counsellors should be prepared to listen. They need to be open-minded and able to offer empathy towards their clients. This doesn't mean they are super human or without normal emotional responses when they feel challenged, but the aim in learning to be a counsellor is to be fully aware of one's personal feelings and reactions and identify them where they could be improved.

When I returned to the university centre after some weeks of illness, I found no welcome from the vast majority of the students on my course, and the tutors. Where was their **congruence**? All they did, was share a form of pack mentality and a belief (shamelessly fostered by the tutors who wouldn't mark my work) that I was affecting more erudition than I had.

Much of the work of a person-centred counsellor must be related to honesty, and minus self-awareness it's a poor therapeutic process. The counsellor must tune in to his or her own thoughts and feelings, and be acutely aware of the need to make every effort to comprehend or at least empathise with the client. So, congruence is a word that gets bandied about and trainees and tutors set great store by it.

Unfortunately, without a good understanding of psychodynamic theories to thoroughly support their beliefs, a counsellor who works primarily in the person-centred model will make mistakes. In forty-minute process groups, learners sit on chairs placed in a circle or semi-circle, chat and try to understand their own responses to others. Such sessions are thought to be helpful, even essential, but speculative efforts cannot possibly create the same learning curve as expert tuition from erudite course leaders. This failure becomes significant when, at a later date, students are permitted to counsel clients equipped mainly with their own guesswork.

Worse, after qualifying with just a diploma for a couple of years' attendance and practise, they may not have been well guided and a great many of their outcomes are questionable. They might make assumptions about their abilities and therefore their personal value, and those assumptions may be flawed.

It's usual for a person-centred counsellor to be told they must identify any client who causes them to feel challenged and, in that instance, it's thought they might wish to explain to the client they are not the right person to offer them therapy. This is important where a subject might arise and be intolerable for the counsellor (for instance, I couldn't listen to someone who thoroughly disliked animals discussing their views) but the point is missed by many learners and tutors. It's also important where the subject is just too complicated for the counsellor to grasp. They must confess!

However, I have met counsellors who are reluctant to acknowledge their personal difficulties. Instead, they try to battle through the counselling process with a client who challenges them, whether that happens deliberately or not. The very existence of a client who is profoundly different from the counsellor, can be a challenge in itself.

If the contents of this book have interested you, please let me know!
Lisaskeet@live.co.uk

Review Requested:
We'd like to know if you enjoyed the book. Please consider leaving a review on the platform from which you purchased the book.

Lightning Source UK Ltd.
Milton Keynes UK
UKHW012324280222
399366UK00010B/653/J